A
MOST SATISFACTORY MAN

The Story of Theodore Brevard Hayne,
Last Martyr of Yellow Fever

For Peter Wood,
   A most satisfactory
man,

   [signature]

November 1996

A
MOST SATISFACTORY MAN

The Story of Theodore Brevard Hayne,
Last Martyr of Yellow Fever

CHARLES S. BRYAN

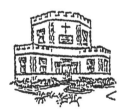

Published for the
WARING LIBRARY SOCIETY
MEDICAL UNIVERSITY OF SOUTH CAROLINA
CHARLESTON, SOUTH CAROLINA
by
THE REPRINT COMPANY, PUBLISHERS
SPARTANBURG, SOUTH CAROLINA
1996

An original publication, 1996
The Reprint Company, Publishers
Spartanburg, South Carolina 29304

ISBN 0-87152-496-1
Library of Congress Catalog Card Number 95-50693
Manufactured in the United States of America

 The paper used in this publication meets the requirements of American National Standard for Information Sciences—Permanence of Paper for Printed Library Materials, ANSI Z39.48-1984.

Library of Congress Cataloging-in-Publication Data

Bryan, Charles S.
    A most satisfactory man : the story of Theodore Brevard Hayne,
last martyr of yellow fever / Charles S. Bryan.
        p.   cm.
    "Published for the Waring Library Society, Medical University of
South Carolina, Charleston, South Carolina."
    Includes bibliographical references and index.
    ISBN 0-87152-496-1
    1. Hayne, Theodore Brevard, 1898-1930.   2. Yellow fever—Africa,
West—History.   3. Physicians—South Carolina—Biography.
4. Physicians—Africa, West—Biography.   I. Waring Library Society.
II. Title.
RA644.Y4B79   1996
610'.92—dc20
    [B]   95-50693
                                                                CIP

For the Hayne Family

Contents

Chapter   Page

    Acknowledgements   ix

    Prologue: Epitaph in a Country Churchyard   1

1   "Not Like His Father"   7

2   Young Malariologist   19

3   To Beard the Lion   43

    Illustrations   *following page* 54

4   "A Most Satisfactory Man"   55

5   Diagnosis Yellow Fever   85

6   Coming Home   115

    Epilogue: "That's Theodore's Car"   127

    Notes   131

    Index   159

Acknowledgements

This is the story of a forgotten investigator who studied a nearly forgotten disease. Two collections of unpublished materials allow me to tell it: personal correspondence shared by relatives of Theodore Hayne and documents at the Rockefeller Archive Center, North Tarrytown, New York.

For most of the personal correspondence, I am indebted to Susan Davis Darby and Margaret Foster Curtis. Other Hayne relatives who provided letters, photographs, or memories include Theodore Brevard Hayne, IV, Susie Stephenson Hayne, Frances Hasell LaBorde, Theodore Hayne Darby, John C. Foster, J. Preston Darby, Bitsy Curran Foster, Hamlin Beattie, III, and Julia Courtenay Campbell. Two of Hayne's sisters, Frances Hayne Hasell and Lillah Adams Hayne, told stories that illustrated his personal qualities, as did William Weston, Jr., and Laura Jervey Hopkins. Julian C. Adams permitted me to rummage through the attic at Wavering Place, resulting in finds that clarified several aspects of Hayne's checkered college career.

I am indebted to the staff of the Rockefeller Archive Center and especially to Harold Oakhill and Melissa A. Smith for invaluable help during my visit and subsequently. The diary kept by Henry Beeuwkes, Hayne's superior at Yaba, enabled me to correlate personal letters with events in Nigeria. I also thank Nancy J. Hulston and Barry Bunch of the University of Kansas, Kansas City; Elizabeth Tunis, Margaret Kaiser, and Peter B. Hirtle of the National Library of Medicine, Bethesda, Maryland; Elizabeth Y. Newsom and W. Curtis Worthington, Jr., of the Waring Historical Library at the Medical University of South Carolina, Charleston; Allen H. Stokes, Jr., of the South Caroliniana Library at the University of

South Carolina, Columbia; and Colin Rowe of the Partnership House Library, London. I am indebted to the Rockefeller Archive Center for permission to reproduce photographs and quotations from manuscript materials; to The Citadel Archives for permission to reproduce two illustrations from *The Sphinix* (1920); and to the Southern Medical Association for permission to reproduce four illustrations that appeared in my article on Theodore Hayne (*Southern Medical Journal* 86 [1993]: 710-715).

Although this book was largely written in the traditional style of the solitary scholar glued to his personal computer, many persons helped along the way. Todd L. Savitt read the first draft and made numerous suggestions, including the viewpoint that Hayne might be seen as representative of his generation's physician-scientists. Edward H. Beardsley's close perusal of the second draft was immensely helpful. Thomas A. Monath, Theodore E. Woodward, John A. Kerr, Jr., and Scott B. Halstead offered useful perspectives on the era and its personalities. I thank Chandlee Bryan for research assistance; W. Curtis Worthington, Jr., Elizabeth Y. Newsom, Jane McC. Brown, and Joy Drennen for editorial suggestions; Dianne Carr for copy editing; Mimi Ackerman for proofreading; and Susan Dugan for help with manuscript preparation. Finally, I thank the many people who encouraged me—especially my wife, Donna, who assisted me at the Rockefeller Archive Center, criticized the manuscript, and supported its completion.

Prologue
Epitaph in a Country Churchyard

*After all, faith is not belief in spite of evidence, but life in scorn of conse-
quence—a courageous trust in the great purpose of all things and press-
ing forward to finish the work which is in sight, whatever the price may
be.*
— Kirsopp Lake, 1920

*Persistent endeavor by the members, present and past, of the Interna-
tional Health Division engaged in the study and control of yellow fever
has yielded basic knowledge of the nature of this disease which is of the
highest importance. These results have been gained in the face of immi-
nent danger, throughout years marked by the sacrifice of brilliant lives.*
— John D. Rockefeller, Jr. and Max Mason to
Dr. Henry Beeuwkes, May 25, 1932

The history of medicine holds a special place for those who
died young but whose uncommon qualities and idealism continue to inspire us. There was, for example, James Jackson, Jr. (1810-
1834), son of a famous Boston physician, who as a medical student
meticulously recorded cases of cholera and gave the first account of
hereditary emphysema, only to die of dysentery shortly after receiving his diploma. There was John Y. Bassett (1805-1851) rescued from
anonymity by William Osler in his essay, "An Alabama Student."
Bassett left his family and practice in Huntsville to study medicine in
Paris only to die of tuberculosis shortly after his return. There was
Francis Weld Peabody (1881-1927), the young Harvard professor
nearing the prime of life who, dying of cancer, gave to an audience of
medical students and to posterity those stirring words, "The secret of
the care of the patient is in caring for the patient." And there have
been martyrs of the diseases they studied, such as Daniel A. Carrión
(1858-1885, who died of bartonellosis), Jesse W. Lazear (1866-1900,

1

of yellow fever), and Howard Taylor Ricketts (1870-1910, of typhus). My purpose is to nominate for inclusion in this select group Dr. Theodore Brevard Hayne (1898-1930), of Congaree, South Carolina.

Before 1987, I had never heard of Hayne. In May of that year, the Centers for Disease Control reported that three health care workers had acquired the "AIDS virus" (the human immunodeficiency virus or HIV) when infected blood touched their skin or mucous membranes. Their cases differed from others in that there had been no cuts, accidental injections, or needlestick injuries—just contact with blood.[1] Concern often bordering on hysteria rippled through America's medical communities, causing an epidemic of meetings. Everyone wanted to talk and talk and talk about AIDS.

On their minds were such issues as whether physicians had the right to refuse to care for HIV-infected patients. If they did, what about nurses and other health care workers? Did HIV-infected patients have a duty to inform health care workers of their status? Did HIV-infected health care workers have a duty to inform their patients? Should HIV-infected health care workers be allowed to continue their practices? Should all patients, all health care workers, or even all citizens be tested for antibodies to the virus? As an infectious disease specialist in a medium-sized Southern city, I had been in the thick of these and other controversies and, before long, had AIDS burnout.

Before AIDS, infectious disease specialists were often regarded as curiosities even in the medical community. Suddenly, we were in demand. I chaired two AIDS task forces, spoke to numerous organizations, and fielded such questions on call-in radio and television shows as "Can you get AIDS from mosquitoes?" While some of the questions were laughable, the concern was valid. Earlier that year, a nurse working in our hospital's emergency room had been tragically infected by the deadly virus. An unusually caring person, she had volunteered to draw blood from an HIV-positive dialysis patient. A freak accident caused the patient's blood to be injected into her tissues. She had already been accepted to our medical school, and her enrollment would prompt still another round of meetings fraught with thinly-veiled hysteria.

It was in this context that a diversion led to the story that follows. An invitation to review the history of the Columbia Medical Society gave me an excuse to escape during lunch hours to the archives of the South Caroliniana Library. Slowly but surely, the nine dusty volumes revealed how each generation of physicians had aspired to lofty ideals only to regress when their basic security needs were threatened. The project was fun, and the pace quickened. Then one day, the turning of another browning page introduced me to Hayne.

The story began innocuously enough. "Theodore Brevard Hayne was born August 3, 1898, at Blackstock, S.C., at which place part of his boyhood days were spent. He was the eldest son of Dr. James A. Hayne and Fannie Thorn Hayne. . . ." Unlike most of the others, this obituary was neatly-typed, double-spaced. Suddenly, it became clear why someone had taken such pains. Leaving the library, I headed east, past the site of Sherman's headquarters, past the ruins of General Wade Hampton's mansion, out the Sumter Highway, and down a country road to a sign that read, "The Episcopal Church Welcomes You." The turn-off promised little more than fields, woods, nondescript houses, and—one assumed—a country church. The neat, newly-white wooden church stood in a clearing with no sign of life. I soon found the tombstone and read the inscription: "THEODORE BREVARD HAYNE, M.D. DIED OF YELLOW FEVER IN LAGOS, NIGERIA, WEST AFRICA. INTERMENT AUG. 24, 1930. GREATER LOVE HATH NO MAN THAN THIS, THAT HE LAY DOWN HIS LIFE FOR HIS FRIENDS."

The HIV-positive medical student was present at my address to the Columbia Medical Society that fall. She smiled knowingly at Hayne's story. She later won the admiration of a community by completing four years of medical school and six months of residency before succumbing to the disease. There is no clear parallel between AIDS and yellow fever; they are different diseases for different times. But health care workers and researchers still need the same set of virtues—especially, courage. Her case had been an exception: the risk of acquiring AIDS from a needlestick injury is small. Hayne, on the other hand, had assumed a risk calculated by his peers to be without precedent in the history of medicine.

Just two months after his wedding in 1930, Hayne had returned for a second tour of duty in Nigeria to assume an especially dangerous task. He took charge of the mosquitoes and monkeys infected with the yellow fever virus at a small research compound run by the Rockefeller Foundation. Five Rockefeller Foundation researchers had already died of the disease—five of a full-time work force that never numbered more than 27 investigators. Hayne knew that infected mosquitoes escaped from time to time from the netting that contained them. He knew that one bite could be his death warrant and that he could even acquire the disease without knowing that he had been bitten. Ultimately, that was what happened. He was the last yellow fever investigator to die of the disease. A vaccine became available the next year. Theodore Brevard Hayne, 1898-1930. Courage.

During the next two years, I mentioned Hayne's story in my talks about AIDS and in two editorials for the state medical journal. That seemed to be the end of it. Then, I met a younger man named Theodore Brevard Hayne. Ted Hayne put me in touch with relatives who shared numerous photographs and unpublished letters, most of them from Hayne in West Africa to his mother. The letters revealed an energetic young man who loved life, people, cars, and the pursuit of mosquitoes and the diseases they cause. There were also letters written about Hayne by contemporaries. These revealed a self-confident, well-motivated, and unusually likable young man who seemed to have been a great favorite of all who knew him. Soon, I wanted to learn everything I could about him. The path led to the Rockefeller Archive Center in Pocantico Hills, New York, where a diary kept by Hayne's superior at Lagos, Dr. Henry Beeuwkes, surrendered the story behind the story, the story of what was happening at the Rockefeller research compound at Yaba, the story of mosquitoes, monkeys, and cutting-edge research. Hayne seemed to be on the threshhold of a significant career in public health when he met his untimely fate.

Hayne's story, I concluded, deserved wider appreciation for at least three reasons. First and most obvious is the lesson in courage, which can be understood as the overcoming of obstacles in order to achieve a socially-desirable goal through the use of both moral and practical reasoning. Moral reasoning involves analysis of the risk and a decision to proceed; its facilitating virtue is altruism. Practical reasoning involves analysis of the problem and formulation of action steps; its facilitating virtue is persistence.[2] Hayne clearly knew the danger of yellow fever. He reputedly told his father that he was going back to Nigeria because the researchers were "doing more than dying there."[3] Having made the commitment, he focused on the tasks at hand, attending to such details as the mesh size of the mosquito cages, knowing all the while the danger.

A second reason to tell Hayne's story is his representation of a fine type of physician-investigator perhaps more common to his era than our own. With Hayne at Yaba were other young men with similar backgrounds and aspirations. Henry Kumm, like Hayne, had left a new bride behind when he sailed from New York. Neil Philip, like Hayne, had worked with the infected mosquito broods and on occasion had been bitten. Austin Kerr, like Hayne, actually acquired yellow fever during his research. Kumm, Philip, and Kerr went on to enjoy long careers and lived to ripe old ages. Of Hayne, the minutes of the Columbia Medical Society recorded that it "was the love of science and not the strains of martial music nor the cheering of his comrades that made Theodore so nobly sacrifice his life, a martyr in the services of mankind fighting an invisible foe."[4] During an era remembered for America's isolationism, these young men went by steamship to fight unfamiliar diseases in unfamiliar lands. All of them took risks; Hayne was the unlucky one.

Finally, there is the personal story of a lovable, energetic young man from a fine old family, secure in his sense of self and place, blessed with a gentle sense of humor, whose practical approach to science and indeed to life compensated for the lackluster record of his formal education. His father, Dr. James Adams Hayne, was a tall, powerful, articulate, colorful, and sometimes controversial figure who dominated public health in South Carolina for nearly four decades. His mother, Fannie Douglass Hayne, the quiet matriarch of a large family, kept a close relationship with her eldest son that offset her husband's detachment. Hayne was also close to his sister Frances (or "Frank"), who married his boyhood friend and college roommate, Philip Gadsden ("Shrimp") Hasell. The supporting cast included two brothers who also became physicians: Isaac (or "Ike") and James ("The Doctor"). Last, there was Roselle, the wife and widow. Standing by Hayne's tombstone that hot July afternoon, I saw a marker next to it—for the stillborn child of the brief marriage. Despite the sad ending, I found the story to be an uplifting chronicle of one man's bright disposition, devotion to a high purpose, and contribution to what many hold to have been one of the United States' finest hours in the field of international health.

1

"Not Like His Father"

J ames Adams Hayne liked a crowd. It was partly for this reason that he went down to Columbia for the rally to protest the sinking of the U.S.S. *Maine* by Spaniards in Havana Harbor. When Adams Hayne recovered from the intoxicating experience, the story goes, he learned that he had just volunteered for the United States Army.[1] He would have to leave his wife, pregnant with their first child. This would be the first of a series of home-leavings that transformed Adams Hayne from a country doctor into a widely-known state health officer. His career would inexorably draw his first child, Theodore, toward three passions: mosquitoes, malaria, yellow fever.

1898—Year of the Mosquito

The South was famous for its fevers. Fevers—arguably more than any other factors aside from the Civil War—distinguished the South from other regions of what is now the United States. Fevers decimated early Spanish and English colonists, dictated the terms of agriculture and commerce, convinced Napoleon to sell the vast Louisiana territory, forced couples to have large families to ensure survivors, and made life always risky and often miserable. Gradually, the fevers were sorted out and given names. None of them were more notoriously Southern than yellow fever and malaria.[2]

Malaria means "bad air." Generations of Southerners blamed it on miasmas (poisonous vapors) that allegedly rose up from the creeks, rivers, inlets, bays, and swamps. The most lethal form of malaria, "blackwater fever," was tamed in part by the introduction of quinine during the 18th century. The milder forms disabled thousands of

Southerners, fueling the myth that they were a lazy people, perhaps even deserving their economic backwardness.

Yellow fever took its name from the characteristic jaundice and its nickname from the quarantine flag, "Yellow Jack," that brought panic to port cities. It struck quickly and without warning, killed up to one-half of its victims, disrupted economies, sparked controversies among physicians and civic authorities, and demanded great courage of those who stayed behind to care for the sick. Epidemics of yellow fever became both more common and more severe in the Southern port cities as their populations increased after the Revolution.[3] Yellow fever fueled the myth that the ante-bellum South was a dark and sinister place, perhaps afflicted by the wrath of God.

To be sure, the South was not unique in the sense that infectious diseases loomed large in its history.[4] Infections had often determined the fate of nations, and at the turn of the 20th century were still the major cause of death in the United States. But the South had more than its share. Thus, when the famous Dr. William Osler addressed the American Medical Association at its 1896 meeting in Atlanta, he chose "The Study of the Fevers of the South." Osler began: "Mankind has three great enemies: fever, famine, and war. And of these, by far the greatest, by far the most terrible, is fever." Osler concluded his address by noting that researchers were uncovering the causes of fever and "the united efforts of many workers in many lands are day by day disarming this great enemy of the race."[5]

The year of Theodore Hayne's birth—1898—might well be called "the year of the mosquito" because of the progress that was made against yellow fever and malaria. Ronald Ross, an Englishman working in Calcutta, showed that the malaria parasite has two separate but mutually-dependent life cycles: one in humans, the other in mosquitoes.[6] A team of Italian workers showed that only *Anopheles* mosquitoes transmitted the disease. The vector (agent of transmission) was now known, as was the basic sequence of events: Human —>*Anopheles* mosquito—>human.

Although mosquitoes were not shown to transmit yellow fever during 1898, Dr. Henry Rose Carter of the United States Public

Health Service came close. Carter studied outbreaks in two north-eastern Mississippi hamlets that consisted of little more than iso-lated plantation houses. He observed that two to three weeks elapsed between the first case of yellow fever in a house and additional cases at the same location:

> The fact that yellow fever is not directly transferable through an environment infected by the patient is due to the fact that the material leaving the patient must undergo some change in the environment before it is capable of infecting another man.[7]

The period required for the change became the "extrinsic incuba-tion." Thus, the sequence of events was: Human—>extrinsic incu-bation (at an unknown location)—>human. All that remained was to locate the site of "extrinsic incubation."

The year 1898 also marked the outbreak of hostilities between the United States and the Spanish Empire. Of the American soldiers who invaded Cuba, 13 died of yellow fever for every one who died from gunfire. General George Sternberg sent a commission headed by Walter Reed to investigate. Carter was put in charge of the quar-antine service in Havana. He kept in touch not only with Reed but also with Reed's young associate, Jesse Lazear. Lazear took up the idea that the *Aedes aegypti* mosquito might be the culprit, an idea seriously proposed in 1881 by a Cuban physician, Dr. Carlos J. Finlay. A mosquito vector was consistent with Carter's demonstration of "extrinsic incubation." The preliminary note by the Reed Commis-sion contained a grim footnote about Lazear, the fourth co-author: "Died of yellow fever at Camp Columbia, Cuba, September 25, 1900."[8] From time to time, it has been suggested that Lazear was on the verge of proof when he allowed a mosquito to bite him in order to make the decisive observations.[9] For his part, Reed was quick to credit not only his co-workers but also Carter: "Your work in Missis-sippi did more to impress me with the importance of an intermediate host than everything else put together."[10] The Reed Commission's work clarified, at least in part, the nature of Carter's "extrinisic incu-bation period." The cycle was: Human—>*Aedes aegypti* mosquito —>human.

The new understanding made possible one of the most dramatic public health demonstrations in the history of the world: the eradication of yellow fever from Cuba by a team led by Colonel William Crawford Gorgas. Gorgas' feat was possible because *Aedes aegypti* is an urban mosquito that breeds almost exclusively in water that is within human control. The Reed Commission had found a strategy but had not found the virus. Much had been done but there was more to learn for "the specific cause of the disease remains to be discovered."[11]

1898—the year of the mosquito. For establishing the role of *Anopheles* mosquitoes in transmitting malaria, Ronald Ross was knighted and received the Nobel Prize. Ross later nominated Finlay and Carter for the Nobel Prize for their parts in establishing a mosquito vector for yellow fever. They didn't get it, but Carter would become—among other things—a mentor for a child born that year, Theodore Brevard Hayne.

Adams Hayne

The Hayne family ranked among South Carolina's most distinguished.[12] Two members are included in today's *Encyclopedia Britannica*: the politician Robert Young Hayne (1791-1839), best known for the 1830 Hayne-Webster debate in the United States Senate, and the poet Paul Hamilton Hayne (1830-1886), prominent among the South's men of letters. The heritage also included Isaac Hayne (1745-1781), a prosperous planter who was the most prominent patriot of the American Revolution to have been hanged by the British. Isaac Hayne had been forced to take an oath of loyalty to the British crown in order to enter Charleston to obtain medical attention for one of his children. Later, when control of the South Carolina lowcountry by the British was less clear, he became an officer in the South Carolina militia. Captured and sentenced to death without a trial, he went to his hanging in front of the Exchange Building in Charleston with a calm dignity.[13] The first Theodore Brevard Hayne (1841-1917) served as an officer in the Confederate Army and commanded an infantry company on April 12, 1861, when shots fired at

Fort Sumter launched the Civil War.[14] In 1868, he married Eliza-beth Adams of a Richland County cotton planting family. Eventu-ally, he became a cotton broker in Greenville. There, his son James Adams Hayne began a circuitous education that included Furman College, The Citadel, the University of South Carolina, the Univer-sity of Virginia, and the Medical College of the State of South Caro-lina, from which he graduated in 1895. Adams Hayne practiced medicine briefly in Greenville and in Athens, Georgia, before set-tling in Blackstock—a small, predominantly rural community in the gently rolling hills near Chester, where people scratched out a living from soil made poor by decades of cotton planting.

Six feet four inches tall, lean, handsome, and gregarious, Adams Hayne was no doubt Blackstock's most eligible bachelor. Fannie Douglass Thorn, who belonged to a large family raised in the coun-try by a widow, began to volunteer to ride the horse into town for the mail.[15] Approaching the doctor's office, she would toss back her straw-berry blond hair and spur the animal into a gallop. The widow Thorn was delighted when Adams Hayne paid a call but anticipated that he had come to see the eldest daughter: "You're here for Adalize?" "No," he replied, "I'm here for Fannie." They were married the same year. Adalize never married.[16]

Like that of most volunteers for the Spanish-American war, Adams Hayne's tour of duty was spent stateside.[17] Mustered out in Novem-ber 1898, he returned to Blackstock where his practice thrived. In 1904, he abruptly left Blackstock for a position with the Examining Surgeon in the Pension Department in Washington, where young Theodore briefly attended school. Eventually, Adams Hayne would be successful in all but monetary terms in numerous roles: public health official, educator, essayist, medical politician, citizen.[18] Many persons would remember him best for a 1920 address entitled "The Rights of the Child," published in *The Journal of the American Medi-cal Association* and considered to have been advanced for his time.[19] Every child, he argued, has the right to be conceived; to be born; to have healthy parents; to have hygienic surroundings; to be breast-fed; to receive good health care; and to "have the best that the resources of any government can command." Adams Hayne obviously liked children and eventually had nine of them. After Theodore came Frances (1900), Lillah (1902), Mary (1904), Isaac (1906), Susan (1909), James Adams (1911), Margaret (1914), and Alicia (1916). Theodore's position as the eldest among many siblings imparted a deep sense of duty and responsibility.[20]

By all accounts, Adams Hayne was a memorable character. Reputed to have had a photographic memory, he could speak eloquently and extemporaneously on just about any subject and often did. There was, for example, the time he solemnly debated another state's health officer on the merits of nightshirts versus pajamas. A grateful nightshirt manufacturer gave him a lifetime's supply. Adding to his notoriety were colorful escapades that often involved drinking and the law. There was, for example, the time in New Orleans that he led a party down to the French Quarter and began to sing in the streets. He was soon directing a large and growing crowd through such refrains as "The Yellow Rose of Texas," "Carry Me Back to Old Virginny," and "Carolina Moon." Bourbon Street proprietors, losing their clientele, summoned the sheriff who told Adams Hayne to leave town.[21]

Theodore Hayne, recalled a contemporary who knew and admired them both, was "not like his father."[22] Although he would share his father's passions and be a man of the out-of-doors, the record indicates that he was closer to his mother. His earliest known letter, written fifteen days after his brother Isaac's birth, suggests that at eight he was already using her nickname, "Fan":

Wed. [December] 26, 1906
My Dear Fan

How are you? We had a nice time yesterday we shot fireworks today. This morning I got a checker board and a pretty plate and a box of paper and a pencil box and a box of candy and a book called "Black Beauty." I went to the Christmas tree when I first got to Blackstock and Sarah Craig gave me a little play watch. When do you want me to come home and is Dady coming over for me. We had a good time and our Christmas tree at

Burns house was fine. Frances and Lillah got a pretty doll and a nice little plate and a box of candy. The little Steeles came to see Frances and Lillah and they had a good time I was in the woods with Mr. Minton getting stove wood and fire wood I am going to the branch in the morning.

> *Your little boy*
> *Theodore Brevard Hayne junior*[23]

(PS) Adalize is sick and in bed.

Young Theodore would soon add to the simple joys of childhood an exposure to the great men of malaria and yellow fever research. His father had taken a position as Medical Officer in the Isthmian Canal Service, Panama, where these diseases ranked high among the issues of the day.

Panama

In 1880, the French had begun to dig a canal across the Isthmus of Panama under Ferdinand de Lesseps, fresh from his triumphant completion of the Suez Canal. By 1898, they had failed—in part due to finances, in part due to engineering problems, and in large part due to disease. They suffered some 50,000 deaths from yellow fever and malaria. Americans resumed the work, expecting that new knowledge might enable them to control malaria and eradicate yellow fever. The physicians, engineers, and scientists who went to Panama for this purpose reflected a "who's who" of authorities on mosquito-borne diseases.

William Gorgas, conquerer of *Aedes aegypti* in Havana, went to Panama in 1904 with the specific charge to protect the workers. Gorgas quickly recruited two men who had been vital to the Cuban campaign: Henry Carter and Joseph Augustin Le Prince. Carter, a Virginian, was an expert in both yellow fever and malaria. Le Prince, a Tennessean, had been Gorgas' sanitary engineer in Cuba and would serve Gorgas as chief sanitary inspector for ten years.[24] In Panama, mosquitoes were attacked by draining, filling land, and destroying larvae by pouring oil on standing bodies of water. The sanitary teams encouraged the use of screens and other measures to keep mosquitoes away from their targets. They captured mosquitoes and studied them, using known research methods and devising new ones. Le Prince and his assistant later wrote a book entitled *Mosquito Control in Panama.*[25]

In 1906, Adams Hayne took the position of superintendent of the sanatorium on Panama's Tobaga Island. The family stayed behind as was their custom. In June 1907, young Theodore wrote his father:

> *My Dear Daddy*
>
> How are you getting along in Panama. Frances stayed in Greenville with Cheremama, and is going to Columbia with Aunt D and Elizabeth & Margaret.
>
> Mr. Minton has been plowing and I went with him and made a pretty little toad-frog town I built a Kings castle and a factory and a lot of houses.
>
> *Your Little Boy*
Theodore[26]

In July, he wrote of financial matters, anticipating what would be a lifelong concern:

> *My Dear Daddy*
>
> How are you. I have gotten the five dollars all right and Fan got the $75 you sent. I went to see Jan Douglas and stayed all day I had a good time. with him. I am going to Blackstock with the mail rider tomorrow We are going to try to have a picknick on my Birthday. I am going to put $4 dollars of my money in the Bank at Blackstock tomorrow. I thank you a milions of times for the five dollars you sent. Frances is crying for Bread and milk and fussing with granny. she is Bad since she came from Greenville. me and Mr. Minter went to the Baptice church to-day we saw Mr. Hickleson and a good many other people we knew.
>
> *Your little Boy*
Theodore[27]

By October, he was thoroughly frustrated with the separation and expressed the desire to go to Panama himself:

My Dear Daddy

> I always forget to write to you. How are you geting along out there? I am having a good time here, but I want to go to Panama and stay with you and eat bananas and oranges, but nobody will take [me]. I am trying to get some one to go with me but I can not get any one to go with me. I went to the fair yesterday by my self and I spent all my money and had to walk home and I got tired walking. It was a man with a white coat on that wun every time, and in the jockeys two diferent men, wun one was a man with a purple jacket on and the other was a man with a white jacket on. I had a sandwitch and coco cola. I will write a longer letter next week.

Your Little Boy
Theodore[28]

He got his wish. The family moved to Panama, and Theodore became at nine the youngest employee of the Panama Canal Commission as a messenger in the Engineering Building.

Although Theodore continued to participate in the usual rites of boyhood, it seems probable that he met Gorgas, Carter, Le Prince, and the other giants of mosquito control. It also seems likely that he began to learn about the subjects that would comprise his life's work: mosquitoes, malaria, yellow fever. Years later, a sister recalled that "Theodore loved mosquitoes-even as a boy."[29]

Wavering Place

The Hayne family moved from Panama back to an ancestral South Carolina home known as Wavering Place, but in a roundabout way. In 1909, Adams Hayne left the Panama Canal Commission to take a commission in the United States Army. He was sent to Fort Assiniboine, Montana, again leaving the family behind in South Caro-

lina. After the birth of a sixth child, Adams Hayne impressed responsibility on his ten-year-old son:

> Your letter received Saturday and Daddy was glad to hear
> from his eldest boy. Just think what a responsibility you now
> have as the eldest son of a family of six. Won't you have a time
> looking after your four sisters—What do you think of your new
> baby sister?[30]

He also reported a match:

> There is [a] little girl out here who I have picked out for a
> sweetheart for you. Her name is Dorothy Chamberlain daugh-
> ter of Lieut. Chamberlain whose wife is from Newberry S.C. . . . .
> You must take good care of Isaac and the new baby and I will
> get you a pony when you come out.[31]

After the family moved to Montana, Theodore reported the life of
an 11-year-old to his grandmother:

> *Fort Assiniboine*
> *Feb. 6 1910*
> *Dear Granny*
>
> I hope you are all well. I have been having a good time skat-
> ing on the pond and irrigation ditches. I skated about twelve
> miles on the irrigation ditches with Lieut Barker. Mary Isaac
> and the baby had their pictures taken in Havre the other day
> and we are sending you all some. Tell Sue to send me the Daniel
> Boone page for boys in the pictorial review. I want to read the
> pieces on it. Tell Adalize to get well and come here and enjoy
> the weather it is not cold at all and not any snow and I hope she
> is getting better. I let one of the big chairs fall on my fingers and
> mashed it bad.
>   Please write soon.
>
>   *Your grandson*
>   *Theodore B. Hayne Jr*[32]

One of Theodore's sisters recalled that he stole a horse at Fort
Assiniboine and rode it into town. Whether for this misdemeanor or

for other reasons, he was sent from Montana to Charleston to continue his education at Porter Military Academy.[33]

The Reverend Anthony Toomer Porter had conceived the idea for the school while visiting the grave of his eldest child who had died of yellow fever. Founded in 1867 for the education of orphans, the school had evolved to include the sons of Charleston families and other pupils "from the country and surrounding islands," some of whom "put sand in their shoes to prevent homesickness." In 1908, the year before Hayne's arrival, two-thirds of the student body had been suspended due to a "Great Rebellion" in which nobody confessed to stealing the school bugle.[34] Of Hayne's record at Porter, nothing is known except that he became fast friends with another pupil from an old South Carolina family: Philip Gadsden Hasell, later known as "Shrimp." In the meantime, Adams Hayne was transferred to Fort D. A. Russell in Cheyenne, Wyoming.

In 1911, Adams Hayne made another transition: he became State Health Officer for South Carolina. The position was relatively new and the appointment largely political, there being few if any formal criteria for public health officials at that time. In South Carolina, as elsewhere in the South, state health departments had emerged largely on account of one disease: yellow fever.[35] Adams Hayne moved his family to an ante-bellum cotton plantation at Congaree, a neighborhood composed mainly of such plantations. Originally called "Magnolia," the plantation was re-named "Wavering Place" allegedly because ownership wavered between the family and the bank. The mansion, three stories high and in the shape of a cube, had been built just prior to the Civil War in the Greek revival tradition typical of its era. It was accessible only by dirt roads and there was no electricity. Although his father was now a public man, young Theodore grew up in the country.[36]

Theodore's sisters would recall that he was "not much of a student." Instead, he showed an aptitude for machinery. He re-built an old Hudson, and, with his cousin, Hamlin Beattie, drove it to Chicago to check it out.[37] He helped construct a small hydroelectric plant to meet the household needs, proudly named The Cedar Creek Power

Company. Spending much of his time in the woods, he became a crack shot. Once, he came home with a bleeding leg and casually told his mother that he had been bitten by a water moccasin but had excised the wound. Eight decades later, a contemporary remembered that young Theodore Hayne "was afraid of nothing."[38]

2
Young Malariologist

As the Panama Canal neared completion, such experts in malaria control as Henry R. Carter and Joseph A. Le Prince renewed their focus on "the malaria problem" of the Southeastern United States. Carter and Le Prince were innovative field workers and were also capable of monumental writing projects.[1] Theodore Hayne had almost surely met them when he was a boy in Panama. At any rate, he would have gained easy introduction through his father's influence. At 16, Hayne began to spend his summers with these giants of malariology. He learned to catch and identify mosquitoes, to know their breeding activity and flight patterns, and to determine when and how they bit humans—sometimes using himself as bait. He would later use these methods in West Africa.

Working with Carter and Le Prince

It was a golden age of malaria research. Knowing that the disease is caused by blood parasites injected by night-feeding female *Anopheles* mosquitoes, health officials could now implement control measures. But many questions remained. Which species of *Anopheles* mosquitoes were important?[2] Where did they breed? When and whom did they bite? What were their flight ranges? What control measures were most cost-effective? These questions needed answers, if only for economic reasons. Carter wrote that the "loss of efficiency caused by malaria in the country of the malarious section of the South is beyond comparison greater than that caused by any other disease, or even by any two or three diseases combined, including typhoid fever and tuberculosis."[3] Such economic importance resulted in political support and funding for control officers and researchers.

In 1912, Carter led an attempt by the U. S. Public Health Service to study malaria systematically.[4] Le Prince and others joined his three-pronged attack: research, education, and practical application of established measures. Under their influence, mosquito-borne diseases became the main focus of Theodore Hayne's life.[5]

Hayne helped Le Prince address the issue of which *Anopheles* species transmitted malaria most frequently. There were three common *Anopheles* species in the South, designated *A. quadrimaculatus* (colloquially, "quads"), *A. punctipennis* ("puncts"), and *A. crucians* ("crucians"). The "puncts" were widespread throughout the Carolinas, yet didn't seem to be important vectors of malaria. Carter wrote that Le Prince and Hayne "found that all of the bites they received on porches, of which they could identify the species (110 in number), were punctipennis." However, the "puncts" did not seem to bite in houses.[6] This study was the first of several known biting experiments in which Hayne used himself as bait.

What Hayne did with Carter is unclear. That he worked directly with the great man is, however, beyond doubt. Carter's daughter, Laura, later wrote:

> Father and I thought the world of him [Theodore Hayne], indeed Father considered him the finest and ablest of the young men with whom he was associated in the latter years of his field work.[7]

Hayne probably became involved in Carter's studies on the effect of impounding water on malaria epidemiology.[8] Dams were being built throughout the Southeast for hydroelectric projects. Would the dams hinder malaria control? Carter determined that mosquitoes thrived around the fallen trees and brush that floated on newly-impounded water. He recommended clearing all growth within proposed lake basins and maintaining clean shore lines. He also found that small fish preyed on mosquito larvae.[9] Carter and others staged public "demonstration projects" to teach the value of such measures as screening, draining, and using larvicides. One participant was Adams Hayne, who wrote about the best way to select towns for the demonstration projects.[10]

Le Prince shared Carter's dual interest in biology and engineering. As early as 1908, he had experimented with ways to trap mosquitoes to study their habits.[11] He also devised a way to determine the flight range of *Anopheles* mosquitoes, a subject on which there was little solid information. The method involved spraying captured mosquitoes with a dilute dye solution using a hand-held atomizer. Researchers liberated the mosquitoes, then tried to re-capture them at various distances from the point of release. They tested the captured mosquitoes for the presence of the dye by placing them on a piece of white filter paper and moistening them with a special solution. Hayne learned this method as a teenager. Later, he would design his own flight experiments in West Africa.

The first major studies of the flight range of American *Anopheles* mosquitoes began in 1914 near Fort Lawn and North Augusta, South Carolina.[12] Hayne participated in studies carried out shortly thereafter in Chester County, during which it was shown for the first time that *Anopheles* mosquitoes could cross a major river. Prior to the experiment, one opinion held that mosquitoes could not cross large streams while another opinion held that mosquitoes could be carried many miles by wind currents. Researchers captured approximately 270 "quads" and 30 "puncts" in houses and barns on the west side of the Catawba, stained them, and released them on the east side of the river. They recaptured three "quads" on the west side—remarkably in the same cabin where they had caught many of the mosquitoes originally.[13] As a 16-year-old technical assistant, Hayne did not receive credit for this work in any publication. However, he could take pride in his contribution. As Henry Carter put it when asked of his own contribution to Walter Reed's discovery, [few]

> scientific discoveries—medical or otherwise—are in their entirety the work of any one man: He who puts the capstone on the completed structure gets—as he should—the credit for it, but the foundation and walls may—and generally have been—built by many hands.[14]

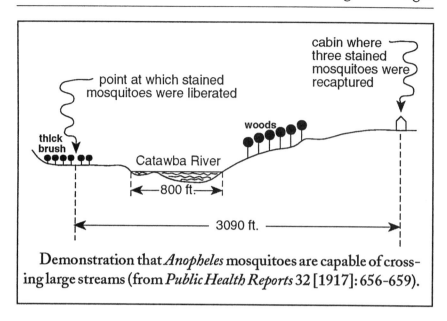

Demonstration that *Anopheles* mosquitoes are capable of crossing large streams (from *Public Health Reports* 32 [1917]: 656-659).

Promoted by his father who had become involved in medical politics, Theodore Hayne's reputation as a young researcher spread widely through the South Carolina medical community.[15]

The Little Salkehatchie Swamp

Young Hayne's word-of-mouth reputation was based in part on an epidemiologic project carried out for a logging company. He was said to have mapped out, single-handedly, South Carolina's Little Salkehatchie swamp.[16] The story was true, but the project was initiated not by an inspired teenager but rather by a law firm. Plaintiffs alleged that the logging activities of The Colleton Cypress Company had promoted *Anopheles* breeding, which in turn had caused cases of malaria. The defense attorneys turned to Henry R. Carter, who in turn suggested that young Hayne could do the work. For $10.00 per day, including expenses, Hayne inventoried the swamp's mosquitoes. He later described his work:

> I made a physical survey of various parts of the Salkehatchie swamp, S.C., near both edges on various spur railroad tracks

and the main track of the Colleton Lumber Co., [an] area adjacent to one of their camps near a causeway crossing, and along the several causeway roads crossing the swamp, at the upper end of the swamp where the lumber has been cut, at places where the lumber had been cut some time ago, and where logs were being taken out at the present time. . . . The Physical survey supplemented by dipping for anopheles larvae gave me a fairly good idea of the mosquito breeding possibilities of this swamp.

He concluded that the logging operations had little or nothing to do with the cases of malaria, since if

every stick of timber and branch that has been felled by the lumber companies and others, and left in the swamp, were removed the number of hiding and protected places for mosquitoes and anopheles development would yet remain so large as to produce sufficient anopheles to reach all houses within a long distance of the swamp, and malaria would probably spread in proportion to the number of persons in the vicinity who were malaria carriers and were accessible to mosquitoes.

Furthermore, another

factor affecting anopheles production that is probably of more importance than the removal of trees and waste left in the water, is the summer periods of dry weather that causes the destruction of the natural enemies of the mosquito larvae. When the small top feeding minnows and predacious insects are destroyed, a much larger proportion of mosquito eggs will develop and a larger number of adult anopheles will be produced, whether trees are felled or not.

Finally:

The vicinity of the swamp is not the only place where malaria has temporarily increased in recent years. The records of malaria in various parts of the country and the others show marked fluctuations in malaria.[17]

Hayne received $200 for his efforts. The defense attorney lamented that Hayne "did not have copies of a map available to designate points on the map for your report" so that it "would have been more easily comprehended."[18] Hayne would always be better at gathering data than at writing up his findings.

He would also be better at studying mosquito-borne diseases than at formal schooling. Needing to continue his education, however, he entered The Citadel in Charleston in 1914 for what would be an extended college career.

Happy Cadet

The Citadel, a military boys' school which had assumed the name of the arsenal in which it was originally housed, stressed military training, discipline, and tradition. Citadel men took pride that members of the Corps of Cadets had fired at the *Star of the West* as she entered Charleston Harbor to reinforce Fort Sumter on January 9, 1861. Applicants were required to be "physically fit for military duty."[19] Campus life revolved largely around a system of merits and demerits. Merits were given for one week's perfect conduct. Well-shined shoes and immaculate rooms were major desiderata. Demerits were meted out for "all the recorded delinquencies" according to "the degree of criminality." Cadets were automatically suspended for 130 demerits in the first year, 150 in the second year, 170 in the third year, or 200 in the fourth year. Events associated with an 1852 yellow fever epidemic illustrate the venerability of the merit-demerit system. After most students fled Charleston on "unauthorized vacation," the Board of Visitors could conceive no greater reward for the nine cadets who stayed at their posts than to remove "all demerit marks up to the time of the Yellow Fever."[20]

Theodore Hayne and his boyhood friend "Shrimp" Hasell entered The Citadel together. They made a bet as to who would finish last. It was close.

Hayne's cheerful disposition resisted the rigorous military code of conduct. Members of The Citadel's class of 1919 gleefully recalled that they had "inherited" him from the class of 1918 and that he "was extremely happy and readily dispensed sunshine, either with his ever-present smile or the melodious notes from his clarinet."[21] He went out for football but was injured, made the track team, and won the marksman's award on the rifle team. His military standing was not helped by such pranks as dropping water bombs on the officer of the day.

Progress in his chosen field, engineering, came slowly. For the 1917–1918 year, Hayne was deficient in his academic work and ranked 197th of 260 cadets in conduct with 135 demerits. The next year, he had the lowest passing grade in the engineering section and ranked 182nd of 350 cadets in conduct with 93 demerits ("Shrimp" Hasell ranked 228th with 127 demerits). But Hayne was not without his own intellectual agenda. In the margin of his textbook on military tactics, he jotted notes on "how to solve direction to fly to compensate sidewinds." He wanted to fly.

He soon got his chance. The outbreak of World War I caught the United States Navy without air power. It had but one aircraft station, 22 training seaplanes, and 38 naval aviators. By the end of the war, there were 42,000 aviation personnel as a result of the buildup. New schools were started, including two on the Pacific Coast: one at San Diego, the other at Seattle. Hayne dropped out of The Citadel and went to Seattle as a student officer.[22]

Hayne's letters offer glimpses of life at the naval school. He wrote his sister Frances:

> We are being worked pretty hard here now, drill most of the time. I'm having a great time learning Radio, semaphone and Fundamentals of Naval Service.
>
> No letter received from home in several days and the camp quarantined. Rain most of the time. Haven't seen the sun but a few times since I've been here.
>
> We had boat drill this afternoon. I had the honored position of stroke oar on the starboard side. Quarantine is still on and I haven't seen all of Seattle.[23]

He wrote his grandmother that he would

certainly be glad when the regular classes start . . . the classes are now fifty each and one graduates every two weeks. Unless the number is increased I shall not leave here until about January 1st 1919.

I haven't been able to leave camp since I've been here on account of the Flu.[24]

Later he reported:

We received a communication from Washington that my company was to be reduced to thirty. Luckily I was not among the twenty names read out to be dropped. . . .

My rating is a temporary one for ground School. It is Chief Quartermaster (Aviation). Corresponding to about sergeant in the Army. When I finish the school shall be commissioned as Ensign.[25]

The war's end abbreviated his flying career. Hayne returned to The Citadel, where the long-awaited senior year would be a trying one.

For the thesis required for his graduation, Hayne chose to write about "The Engineer and Malaria." His first effort was brought to the attention of the school's president, Colonel O. J. Bond, who warned that it was unacceptable for an engineering degree. The essay contained much information about malaria but virtually nothing about engineering.[26] Hayne worried that he would not be allowed to graduate.

He had difficulty sharing this anxiety with his family. "Shrimp" Hasell—who was courting Hayne's sister Frances—took the task upon himself to inform them. Hasell wrote Frances that her brother had trouble concentrating: "There is a big argument in progress in here now. Teddy and Bud Baynard are having an argument about the faculty here." Hasell resumed: "It has taken me two hours to get Teddy started studying but at last he is underway."[27] Later, Hasell confided:

Frank, I'll tell you why Teddy was so grouchy Christmas. He is worried, Frank, worried until he is sick. He is worried about his graduating and then he thinks you and the rest do not care for him.[28]

Possibly, Hayne could not bring himself to share these concerns with his father. Adams Hayne was deeply immersed not only in public health issues but also in medical politics.[29] For whatever reason, Hayne turned to his old mentor, Henry Carter, who gave just the right assurance:

> *Feb 27/[19]20*
> *Dear Theodore*
>
> Engineering is all right. I am an Engineer myself so far as a C.E. degree goes. If I can help you get yours I will be glad to do so.
>
> You have four qualities which should make for success in whatever work you whole-heartedly undertake: integrity; intelligence; persistence & faithfulness to the work undertaken. Whether you [will] make money or not I don't know but you will do good work.
>
> Commend me to your father.
>
> > *Very sincerely,*
> > *Your friend*
> > *H. R. Carter*[30]

Spurred on by such encouragement, Hayne finished. The editors of The Citadel's yearbook, *The Sphinx*, gleefully observed:

> In military, too, "Teddy" has led a varied career. He has held a Cadet office each year; but the acid of demerits ate away his chevrons, so that now he wears a clean sleeve. And, as a result, serious things do not interest "Teddy" much. Give him, rather, the joy of dumping some poor, unfortunate Cadet at night, or the opportunity to deliver a volley of well directed breadballs in the messhall, or the chance to drop a waterbag upon some "tourist"—or even upon the "O.D."—then he is happy. However, he is one of the best fellows in the world, and the reason that he does not graduate a lieutenant, or higher, is not that he lacks ability, but that he loves fun.[31]

For an aphorism, the yearbook's editors looked to Lord Byron:

> Here's a sigh to those who love me,
> And a smile to those who hate;
> And whatever sky's above me,
> Here's a heart for every fate.[32]

The Sphinx bade him farewell:

> "Teddy" is clever, quiet, extremely accommodating, and a
> thoro gentleman. So it is natural that these things, together with
> his handsome physique and polished manners, should have made
> him a favorite with the ladies.
>
> As he leaves us, the Band, the Corps, and the School will feel
> a vacancy here, hard to fill. And, as we part, even tho we know
> that, where'er he goes, success awaits him, we hate to see him
> go.[33]

Sleeping with Pigs

Immediately after graduating from college, Hayne joined the Public
Health Service full-time to do more malaria work. Official notice
came on June 29, 1920 by telegram:

> PUBLIC HEALTH SERVICE WASHINGTON DC
> EFFECTIVE JULY FIRST NOMINATE THEAOR-
> DORE [*sic*] B HAYNE CONGAREE SOUTH CARO-
> LINA TECHNICAL ASSISTANT ONE HUNDRED
> FIFTY MONTH TRAVEL AND PER DIEM THREE
> MONTHS ORDER REPORT FRICKS MEMPHIS BY
> LETTER[34]

More specifically, Hayne was assigned to be a technical assistant to
Dr. Marshall Albert Barber. It is likely that Hayne already knew
Barber, since the latter had been in charge of the hospital base laboratory at Camp Jackson, South Carolina, during 1917-1918. For his
part, Barber was at age 52 on the threshhold of a great second career
as a malariologist.

Although a newcomer to malaria research, Barber was no stranger to the disease. He had been raised in southeastern Kansas, where his "own family had it every autumn."[35] His background included public health, botany, bacteriology, and—most recently—parasitology. He had studied and later taught bacteriology at the University of Kansas and at Harvard. He was somewhat famous for inventing a capillary pipette known as the "Barber micro-manipulator" which allowed bacteriologists to study individual cells.[36] He studied hookworm in the Malay Archipelago and the Fiji Islands. He had become interested in malaria research while working in the Phillipines. As he later explained:

> And why should one stick closely to one sort of microbe? They often hunt human beings in pairs or packs of two or more kinds at once, and it would appear to be logical to hunt them in the same way.[37]

In May 1920, he had became a special expert in malaria research with the U. S. Public Health Service.[38]

However experienced, versatile, and original he might have been, Barber was apparently not an easy man to work for. One Rockefeller staff member who knew Barber wrote a colleague that

> I can understand the difficulty of getting along with him. . . . He has always been a lone worker, and I was surprised to find out how little our staff members got from him except when actually serving him in a capacity close to that of technician.[39]

Perhaps because of his subordinate position, perhaps because of his sunny personality, Hayne seems to have gotten along with Barber famously. Their collaboration would even extend to West Africa.

Hayne and Barber proceeded from Memphis to Stuttgart, Arkansas, center of a rice growing area where malaria was always present and occasionally caused mild epidemics. There they examined school children for malaria parasites.[40] Hayne told his family that in order to learn more about the ways of mosquitoes, he had even slept with pigs. They thought he was joking. He wasn't.

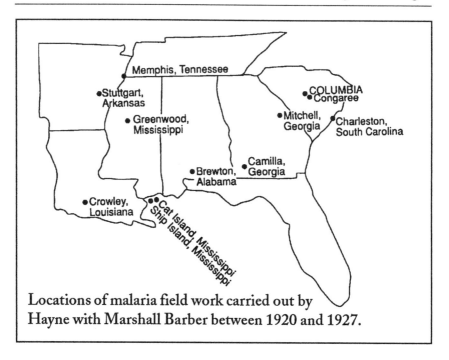

Locations of malaria field work carried out by
Hayne with Marshall Barber between 1920 and 1927.

It had been suggested that domestic animals might buffer humans from mosquitos by offering alternative targets. Barber and Hayne stationed three traps about 100 yards from *Anopheles*-infested rice fields near Stuttgart. The traps were small sheds with dirt floors and slanting wooden roofs. The sides were closed with netting, but space was left open at the bottoms so that mosquitoes could enter:

> The man-baited trap contained nightly one and sometimes two persons (white), rather inadequately protected by a smaller net placed immediately over the bed. The pig-baited trap contained two pigs not protected by net or screen, except in the last experiment. A control trap, containing no source of blood, was placed midway between the other two traps. Both men and pigs remained all night in the traps, and the mosquitoes were collected at dawn.

Between August 5 and August 8, 1920, Barber and Hayne caught 457 mosquitoes in the man-baited trap and 494 in the pig-baited trap. Only 93 mosquitoes drifted into the control trap. Next, they put the pigs in a screened box that they then placed in the former control trap. They left the original pig trap empty as a new control:

> The man-baited trap contained one person. Unfortunately this experiment was somewhat marred by a thunderstorm with a high wind, to which the man-baited trap was somewhat more exposed than the other traps.

Thus while domestic animals might indeed buffer humans in that they could "satisfy mosquitoes that otherwise might have fed on man," there was little support for the idea that livestock specifically protected humans from malaria.[41]

It may have been during this period that Hayne experienced a severe attack of malaria, from which he recovered. Hayne returned to South Carolina, where he did some more malaria work in November and December of 1920. After Christmas leave, he re-joined Barber at Camilla, Georgia. There, they made a discovery that secured for both of them a place in the history of malaria research: the efficacy of Paris green as a larvicide.

Paris Green

Destroying larvae is central to mosquito control. The standard method throughout the malarious sections of the world was to float oil on the surface of water. This practice was cumbersome, unaesthetic, and potentially harmful to other forms of life. However, it was widespread. In 1923, for example, a citizen of Bottineau, North Dakota, wrote the Bureau of Public Health in Washington, D.C.:

> With 10,000,000 automobiles in the country, there must be millions of gallons of crank-case oil wasted every year. This oil could be saved and used to put on pools of stagnant water and thus kill misquitoes [sic]. I hope you will be able to give this some publicity.[42]

An alternative method was badly needed.

A French investigator had tried poisoning the larvae with a substance known as trioxymethylene. Barber and Hayne experimented with numerous compounds in search of a more potent and practical chemical larvicide. Perhaps acting "on a tip from someone in New Orleans,"[43] they found that Paris green, an arsenic compound, killed larvae at extremely low concentrations that had little or no effect on other marine life. In their article on "Arsenic as a Larvicide for Anopheline Larvae," Barber and Hayne explained the rationale:

> These [mosquito] larvae lie at the surface of the water, and in feeding turn the head halfway around into such a position that the feeding brushes carry to the mouth any particles lying on the surface-tension layer of the water. The larvae swallow all floating substances that are small enough to enter the mouth easily, and are quite indifferent as to whether these are food or poison. No bait of any kind is required to make these larvae eat anything that is offered to them.[44]

Paris green was extremely cheap. When packed in 300-pound barrels, it cost only about 22 cents per pound. Paris green could also be diluted with any inert dust, such as fine sand, rotten wood dust, or road dust. A dilution of one part of Paris green to 100 parts of dust made a suitable mixture. Thus diluted, Paris green had a wide margin of safety. Barber and Hayne reported that "we have used no precautions other than to stand to the windward of the dust cloud—the place where one would naturally stand in distributing the dust—and we have experienced no harmful results whatever."[45] They predicted that it would be widely used. It was.

Paris green became the larvicide of choice throughout the malarious sections of the world for about a quarter of a century—until the introduction of DDT.[46] The dust was thrown onto water by hand, dispersed by various types of blowers, and even released from airplanes. For many years, a touched-up photograph of young Theodore Hayne dispensing Paris green from a flat-bottomed boat hung in the parlor at Wavering Place. Hayne's part in the discovery brought him early recognition within the community of malariologists.

In August 1921, Hayne resigned from the Public Health Service to spend "a few days at home before re-entering school."[47] His hope was to go to medical school. However, there was no money.[48] Therefore, he re-joined the Public Health Service in January 1922 and went to Brewton, Alabama, to help Barber with "the establishment of a field laboratory." Further studies were carried out on Ship Island and Cat Island off the coast of Mississippi with the conclusion that Ship Island might be "an ideal site for the further investigation of mosquito control by use of Paris green."[49] However, there were many more questions to be addressed.

What was the range and life expectancy of *Anopheles* mosquitoes in the Arkansas rice country? Barber and Hayne found that mosquitoes could live up to 25 days in midsummer and could spread for about a mile from the rice fields in open country.[50] To what extent did mosquitoes survive during the winter? They found that control measures were needed throughout the year.[51] Could the the sex distribution of mosquitoes be used to predict the location of a breeding site, as was commonly thought? They disproved this notion.[52] Although Hayne was no doubt encouraged by the success of these studies, he realized that a higher degree would be necessary if he were to advance his career. He resigned from his $1800.00 per year position and on September 23, 1923, entered The Medical College of the State of South Carolina.

Medical School

At that time, the Medical College in Charleston was a struggling institution that bore little resemblance to the fine tertiary care center it was later to become.[53] There was only a small full-time faculty in the basic sciences, and the clinical faculty was mostly part-time. Formal requirements for admission consisted of "graduation of an approved four-year high school, and satisfactory completion of two years of college work." Adams Hayne held the rank of Professor of Public Health Administration at the Medical College, in which capacity he drove down periodically from Columbia to lecture to the fourth-year class. Although Theodore Hayne might turn to his father for advice and guidance, Adams Hayne could offer little financial assistance even though tuition was only $150 per year. Henry R. Carter loaned Hayne money for tuition and expenses.

Few details survive of Hayne's sojourn through medical school. He lived with the Hasell family at 64 Warren Street, the relationship between the two families having been cemented by "Shrimp" Hasell's engagement to Frances Hayne (they were married on November 24, 1924). He later advised his younger brother, Isaac: "If you take some notes on all that Dr Philips [William Fowke Ravenel Phillips] tells you in anatomy you will never regret it. You won't appreciate what good stuff he does teach until you are finished at the medical college."[54] Nearing graduation, he confided to a friend: "The same old grind continues here but occasionally we see some unusual case or note some unusual change in a patient on the wards which compensates for the hours of lecture work. Didactic work is not my hobby."[55]

His favorite hobby was fixing cars, for which he would always be in demand. Thus, Fannie Hayne indicated that Theodore was coming home "to fix up Anthony's Scripps Booth for him, he let the water freeze in his and busted his engine so he bought our old Scripps from us and he wanted Theo to fix it for him."[56] Hayne wrote his brother, Isaac, of his continued devotion to younger siblings and ailing automobiles:

64 Warren St
Charleston, SC
March 25, 1924

Dear Ike,

I hear that your report was pretty good. Am sure glad to hear it. Was up at the new Citadel Sunday with Shrimp and everything looked fine. The alumni building has a fine 22 gallery rifle range. They didn't go to Mt Pleasant for the weeks practice as usual this year on account of the ferry's not running.

Ive been wondering just what course youve been thinking of taking when you go to college. Whether you expect to be a Doctor, Civil Engineer, Chemical, Electrical, Mechanical, or

Sanitary engineer, Journalist, Lawyer, Chemist, etc etc. Write me what course youve been thinking of and Ill tell you all I know about each and find out much more to tell you. Will also find out the best place to take the work you want most. Fan said you had talked of Farming. Whatever is to be your chosen profession will require its particular special studies. Its important to be thinking this all over in your spare time and ask some of your professors about it. They will be glad to help you.

What time does your school close? When does the Spring vacation begin?

Almost is running like a scared rabbit now. Just needs the tin on the dash. We found the wire trouble & she steps out now.

Think Ive sold Shrimp's stripped Republic truck for $40. Man is [to] be back later this week.

Never did get Anthony's car to run. Will work some more when I go home again.

Well write me a long letter & tell about yourself.

Your brother
Theodore

P.S. Who's your girl?[57]

During medical school, Hayne continued to devote his summers to malaria research with Marshall Barber. They found that water hyacinth, a favorite ornamental plant, encouraged mosquito breeding.[58] They confirmed that *Anopheles quadrimaculatus* ("quads") was the most important vector of malaria in the South, although other species might have had minor roles.[59] And they obtained evidence that malaria was finally beginning to decline in the rural South. It was still present in the rice prairies of Louisiana and Arkansas, but deaths were rare and conditions were becoming more favorable for agriculture.[60] Random surveys on plantations in the delta counties of Mississippi indicated that about five percent of the population carried malaria parasites, compared with 20 percent nine years earlier.[61]

Malaria was declining, but nobody knew exactly why. Possibilities

included the specific control measures and changing agricultural practices. Marshall Barber, who considered malaria to be a "disease of
defective civilization," was "inclined to give the greater credit to
screens, quinine, and improved medical treatment."[62] In 1926, the
summer before his senior year in medical school, Hayne conducted
his own survey in the Mississippi Delta. He undertook a house-to-
house survey of 1,859 persons belonging to the "renter class" of both
races on the cotton plantations. He made notes on the living circumstances, asked who was sick, and obtained blood samples. He confirmed that malaria was now uncommon and that economic improvement was at least partly responsible. More than one-half of the houses
had some kind of screening. Automobiles were found in 42 percent
of the yards. Hayne ended his paper with a wry observation that the
"large percentage of automobiles per family does not necessarily indicate a highly mobile population since many of the automobiles were
incapable of locomotion."[63]

With the publication of his paper in the *Southern Medical Journal*,
Hayne had demonstrated his ability to carry out research independently.

Internship in Panama

In 1927, Hayne graduated from medical school on schedule in a
class of 32 students, all but two of whom were native South Carolin-
ians.[64] It was then the custom to serve a one-year rotating internship.
Hayne chose Ancon Hospital (later Gorgas Hospital) at Ancon, Canal
Zone, to which he was appointed with "the marvelous compensation
of $75 per month & transportation from New York."[65] Arriving in
Panama, he found the hospital to be "a beautiful building and all
equipment very modern. . . . The view of the city & bay from our
location on the side of Ancon hill is truly beautiful."[66] Indeed the
hospital, originally built by the French Canal Company in 1883 on
the slopes of Ancon Hill, was considered by many persons to be among
the most beautiful medical facilities in the world.

At one time, the hospital also ranked among the world's most dangerous on account of yellow fever. Under the French, it had been
operated by the Sisters of St. Vincent de Paul, who also had a pen-

chant for ornamental gardening. To protect their flower beds from leaf-cutting umbrella ants, the sisters surrounded the beds "with a concrete curb grooved to hold a ribbon of water." *Aedes aegypti* mosquitoes thrived in these troughs, gained easy entrance to the adjacent unscreened hospital wards, and thus caused many and perhaps most of the 1,200 deaths from yellow fever that occurred at the hospital between 1883 and 1889.[67] The French did not know, of course, that yellow fever was transmitted by mosquitoes. It was therefore especially fitting that Ancon Hospital was re-named Gorgas Hospital after the death of Gorgas, conquerer of yellow fever in Panama.

Hayne began his internship with a surgical rotation, writing a friend that he was spending "most of the time assisting in the operating room."[68] He later wrote his mother that he had

> been busy in the eye ear nose and throat department for the last week but dont think that I would prefer this branch of medicine for making a living altho it is said to be very remunerative. Have seen and assisted in tearing out a number of tonsils and adenoids but dont think the surgical technique is as good as that employed in the general surgical department.[69]

He later confirmed his decision to his father despite the apparent improvement in his own surgical technique:

> Dont think the Eye Nose & Throat work appeals to me tho thus far Ive removed ten pair of tonsils under local anesthetic and one under general without fatalities or severe hemorrhage. The uvula was intact in all cases tho often somewhat oedematous after. The ptyergium operation could still see after my brutal surgery and the peritonsillar abscess hasn't found it necessary to ligate the jugular vein yet but nature's ability to repair trauma should be given entire credit for the results.[70]

Hayne had similar reservations about the medicine service:

> Dont think I am learning as much medicine in this service as I should like. The medical officers of the army, here, in general, are not particularly good diagnosticians. They certainly make use of all laboratory aids ever devised but don't seem too good at

giving proper weight to findings after they get thru. Im the goat
of course on the laboratory work [and] must do all of the blood
smears, wassermans, etc etc as well as take admission histories
and do physicals on all patients. Theres so much paper work
charting and laboratory tests & so little done for [the] patient.
It leaves little time for me to observe cases and read up anything
about the various diseases.[71]

There was, however, time to enjoy the experience of being a young
person in Panama. The interns did not receive salaries but nevertheless found

> something to do almost every night. Its either a boat ride in the
> bay, a hike to the top of Ancon Hill, a dance at the Century
> club, or a swim in the large Balboa pool.[72]

Hayne found time for a hunting trip on which he and another physician "killed about 20 crocodiles saw a group of monkeys in the jungle
and admired the various birds which were flying about."[73] He up-
dated his father on Panamanian night life:

> The Initropale continues an attractive place tho Ive been there
> only three times since I came down. Kelleys Ritz attracted the
> internes at first but was found to be too expensive. The Century
> Club continues to be the meeting place when away from the
> hospital but when visitors come down who have some idea of
> mixed drinks the International Hotel is chosen because the mix-
> tures there are the best.[74]

He reassured his mother not to

> worry about my running with any fast set down here. The only
> associates that we have are the internes and nurses. The forms
> of amusements are two or three dances a month at the Century
> Club and movies in Panama.
>
> My girl has gone to the states on a two months vacation so
> that I haven't anyone to go to Taboga with. Thats the expensive
> trip.[75]

Except for such references to "my girl," Hayne's letters provide little information about his courtship of Anne Roselle Hundley, a nurse at Ancon Hospital who is remembered as "a beautiful brunette with dark eyes."[76]

Perhaps there was little of an extravagant nature to report. Anticipating the completion of his internship, Hayne noted that there were not

> but about seven more months when I shall have to begin making some money to pay back my numerous debts. Havent decided exactly what to do but suppose that I shall take the first sure salaried job that will bring in the largest amount of money for a year or so.[77]

In December, he wrote his father that he was

> expecting to begin negotiations about Jan 1st with I.H.B. [International Health Board of the Rockefeller Foundation], United Fruit and even the P.H.S. Dr Barber still has some work to do. They stopped over on the way to Costa Rica and spent the afternoon on this side with me.[78]

On January 15, 1928, Hayne applied formally to the International Health Board of the Rockefeller Foundation:

> About July 1st, 1928 I shall complete a year's internship at Ancon Hospital and will be desirous of obtaining more permanent work. During eleven summers previously I was employed by the U. S. Public Health Service on field investigation of malaria as an assistant to Drs. Carter and Barber.
>
> I want to know what work may be obtained with the International Health Board at this time.[79]

Although Hayne did not advertise his experience, his work with Barber was obviously known at the Rockefeller Foundation. Dr. John A. Ferrell replied:

> We were glad to have your inquiry of the 15th and we would welcome an opportunity to discuss with you your plans and possibilities for service with the Foundation. The program to which

we are committed should offer you an opportunity to capitalize the exceptional training and experience you have had in malaria work.[80]

Ferrell suggested that Hayne be a special staff member initially, and that his status might be changed to that of regular member if after "at least a year it should be mutually agreeable." Hayne responded that this condition was satisfactory, but he added:

> Since much of my previous experience, training, and interest has been in malaria I would like to know where I shall be sent and what work will be expected of me.[81]

Ferrell answered:

> Consideration will be given a little later as to your initial assignment. Doctor Russell may wish to send you to West Africa. As soon as anything definite has been decided we shall let you know.[82]

On March 15, 1928, the Executive Committee of the Rockefeller Foundation approved Hayne's appointment as a special member of the staff of the International Health Division. Dr. Ferrell informed him that he would be assigned to West Africa:

> According to the present plans of Doctor Russell, your appointment will become effective as early after June 15th as you can report for duty and you will be assigned to West Africa to work under the supervision of Doctor Beeuwkes in measures directed to the control of yellow fever. While on this assignment you will receive any special allowances enjoyed by a special member of the staff while engaged in yellow fever work.[83]

Hayne was placed on the "yellow fever mailing list" to receive any new literature "bearing on the situation in West Africa."

Hayne was looking forward to the salaried job, in part for financial reasons. Henry R. Carter, who had loaned him the money for his medical education, had died following a stroke in 1925, and Hayne needed to pay back the loan to Carter's daughter, Laura. In addition, Hayne wanted to help his brother Isaac obtain an education:

Miss Laura Carter wrote me that she had been very sick recently & would like for me to begin paying back the principal as soon as possible as she needed some money. I hope to begin making some money soon. I want to put Ike thru school if I possibly can so that he can go where he wants to.[84]

Meanwhile, his application with the Rockefeller Foundation was progressing on schedule. His senior physician at Ancon Hospital wrote Frederick F. Russell, director of the International Health Board:

The interns each spend six weeks of their year at the Laboratory and Dr. Hayne is just finishing his six weeks with us. He is a tall, fine looking, young man, of good personal appearance and has a pleasing disposition. He will undoubtedly get along well in almost any environment. He attends faithfully to his duties, is studious, and has ability somewhat above the average. During the short time I have known him he has made a very favorable impression and shown no undesirable traits of character.[85]

Before Hayne left for his assignment in West Africa, Russell wrote the director of the Rockefeller research compound at Yaba, near Lagos, Nigeria:

I am sure that you will like Dr. Hayne. Unless something quite unforeseen occurs we expect to take him on our regular staff and to have him as one of our malariologists, since he is a pupil of Dr. Henry Carter and Dr. Marshall Barber, two of the greatest teachers of malaria we have ever had. In fact, Darling was the only other one in their class.

In sending him to you for his first tour of foreign service I am starting what I hope we shall be able to do in the future, that is, to staff the yellow fever work with young well-trained men who will learn their yellow fever in the new school which you and your staff have established in Lagos.[86]

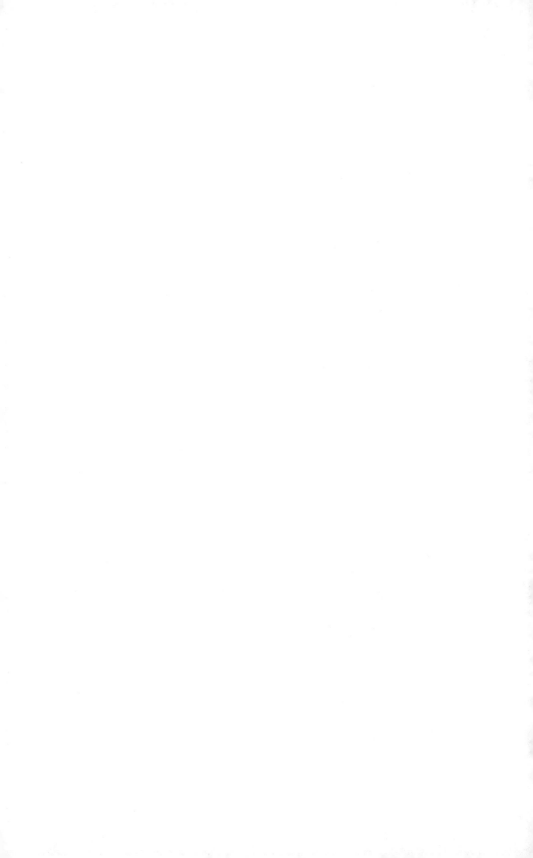

3
To Beard the Lion

Joining the West African Yellow Fever Commission made Theodore Hayne participant to an an international drama orchestrated by the Rockefeller Foundation. In 1916, Rockefeller authorities had concluded that it would be feasible to eradicate yellow fever from the face of the earth and committed huge resources to this aim. In 1933, they concluded that such eradication could not be achieved, at least not during the 20th century. In between these dates, Rockefeller investigators studied yellow fever on two continents, discovered the virus, and devised an effective vaccine. These historic achievements came at great cost—but then, cost was always a feature of yellow fever.[1]

Yellow Fever

Most authorities believe that yellow fever was imported to the Caribbean from Africa by Dutch slave traders, possibly during the 1640s.[2] For nearly three centuries, it tempered human ambitions in the New World as "the terror of the Western Hemisphere." Only land-locked Bolivia escaped. Yellow fever devastated the English and French forces that tried from time to time to displace Spanish dominance in Latin America. The Spaniards suffered equally from what they called *vomito negro* or "black vomit."[3]

The disease spread north from the Caribbean to the port cities of what is now the United States. Between 1668 and 1831, there were 20 epidemics in Philadelphia, 15 in New York, eight in Boston, and seven in Baltimore. The 1793 Philadelphia epidemic was made especially memorable by Dr. Benjamin Rush, who insisted that aggressive bloodletting was the treatment of choice. During the 19th century the disease strengthened its hold on Southern seaports as towns grew into cities. In Charleston, South Carolina, for example, deaths occurred nearly every year. The disease also gripped the Gulf Coast and New Orleans and sometimes travelled up the Mississippi River. The 1878 epidemic reputedly killed eight percent of the population of Vicksburg and 10 percent of the population of Memphis.[4] Yellow fever had replaced smallpox as the premiere cause of terrifying epidemic disease in port cities.

Credit for the first serious implication of mosquitoes in yellow fever usually goes to Josiah Clark Nott, a transplanted native of Columbia, South Carolina, who practiced surgery in Alabama. In 1848, Nott speculated that the disease was of "probable insect or animalcular origin."[5] For years, he argued the case but with little success.[6] Yellow fever claimed four of Nott's own children within a single week even though he had moved his family to "the healthy pine hills" seven miles from Mobile. In 1854, Nott presided over the birth of a child who was named William Crawford Gorgas. Gorgas, who is said to have met his future wife when she was acutely ill with yellow fever, became world famous by showing that Nott was right. To get rid of yellow fever, one must get rid of the right mosquito.

The history of yellow fever during the 20th century is framed by three discoveries. First and best-known is the proof by Walter Reed and his colleagues in 1900 that *Aedes aegypti* is a vector—they thought the only vector.[7] This discovery enabled Gorgas' spectacular campaigns in Cuba and in Panama. Second, Rockefeller Foundation workers transmitted the disease from a human to a rhesus monkey in 1927. This enabled them to isolate the virus and develop a vaccine. Finally, Rockefeller workers showed that mosquitoes other than *Aedes aegypti* could transmit yellow fever. In 1932, an epidemic was reported from Brazil in which *Aedes aegypti* was not the vector. Researchers then realized that there are two patterns of disease transmission. "Urban yellow fever" is transmitted between humans by the domestic mosquito, *Aedes aegypti*. "Jungle yellow fever," on the other hand, is transmitted between monkeys, humans, or both by at least ten species of wild mosquitoes. Jungle yellow fever gives the virus a sanctuary in the remote forests of Africa and South America and makes eradication a difficult task.

Both variants—urban yellow fever and jungle yellow fever—are caused by the same small round virus.[8] The virus attacks primarily the liver, causing jaundice (hence, "yellow fever"). However, it is a generalized infection of many, perhaps most organs including the heart, kidneys, brain and bowel. Between 20 percent and 50 percent of patients who develop jaundice die. It is now recognized that some cases are so mild that the infected person experiences no symptoms whatsoever. People who recover from yellow fever have life-long immunity. However, neither asymptomatic cases nor "jungle yellow fever" were known when the Rockefeller Foundation declared war on yellow fever.

The Rockefeller Foundation Vows to Eradicate Yellow Fever

John D. Rockefeller, deeply impressed by Andrew Carnegie's opinion that "the man who dies rich dies disgraced," had resolved to fund an organization dedicated to "the well-being of mankind throughout the world."[9] The Rockefeller Foundation was formally organized in 1913. Among the first acts was the creation of an International Health Commission (later called a Board and then a Division),[10] to be headed by Wickliffe Rose, a former philosophy professor from Nashville, Tennessee. In 1914, Rose went to Malaya and the Phillippines to study hookworm. He learned that Orientals were concerned that the opening of the Panama Canal might bring yellow fever to the Pacific basin, where it was unknown. Rose discussed the problem with Gorgas. Gorgas replied that yellow fever could be "eradicated from the face of the earth within a reasonable time and at a reasonable cost." Gorgas believed that the Rockefeller Foundation could not undertake a more worthwhile activity.[11]

Gorgas' optimism was based on two assumptions. First, *Aedes aegypti* was the only vector. *Aedes aegypti* is a household mosquito that breeds mainly in human-made water containers. Unlike *Anopheles* mosquitoes, it disdains swamps and similarly difficult-to-reach places. Eradication was therefore relatively straightforward—as Gorgas had shown in Cuba and Panama. Second, "key centers"—towns or cities in which yellow fever persisted year-round—were essential to the survival of the still-unidentified agent of the disease. The reservoir of infected humans in such places allowed mosquitoes to be infected in turn, thereby perpetuating the cycle. Yellow fever would disappear, the reasoning went, if one could just eradicate the "key centers."

On May 26, 1915, a resolution was adopted in New York "that the International Health Commission is prepared to give aid to the eradication of this disease in those areas where the infection is endemic and where conditions would seem to invite cooperation for its control."[12] In 1918, the Rockefeller Foundation formed a Yellow Fever Commission with Gorgas as director. The new commission targeted Guayaquil, Ecuador's major seaport and a hotbed of yellow fever. To Guayaquil was sent Hideyo Noguchi, 43, a brilliant, colorful, outspoken Japanese-born scientist employed by The Rockefeller Institute for Medical Research. Noguchi was an authority on spirochetes and had been the first to show the spirochete of syphilis (*Treponema pallidum*) in the brains of persons demented from the disease. He now resolved to find the cause of yellow fever.[13]

Soon after his arrival in Ecuador, Noguchi isolated a spirochete from the blood of six of 27 patients with yellow fever. Naming the organism *Leptospira icteroides*, he believed that he had found the answer. In retrospect, these patients almost surely had Weil's disease, a severe form of a disease known as leptospirosis that also involves the liver and causes jaundice. Leptospirosis was highly prevalent in Ecuador. The lack of any specific diagnostic test for yellow fever makes Noguchi's mistake understandable. Clinicians frequently could not clearly distinguish yellow fever from other infectious causes of jaundice. Still, only Noguchi's huge reputation explains why so many authorities accepted his answer.[14]

Among the believers was the usually skeptical Henry R. Carter.

Carter had authored the "key center" theory. He reasoned that yellow fever survived because of three factors: human carriers, mosquitoes, and humans who had never had the disease. Bustling port cities such as Quayaquil met all three of these requirements. Small towns with little or no influx of new persons who were susceptible to the disease made it difficult for the virus to perpetuate itself. Carter postulated that yellow fever would disappear spontaneously from small towns and villages once the "key centers" had been cleared. In 1919, he wrote:

> It is facts like these which justify the plan of the International Health Board for the elimination of yellow fever from the earth. ... In my judgment it is entirely feasible. Many places in which yellow fever exists will need but minimal sanitary work to turn the scale against it, and the freeing of one place from yellow fever frequently prevents the infection of some other, making an endless chain of good. Many of the higher forms of life have permanently disappeared from the earth, some in our own times, but this is the first attempt made for this purpose against a micro-organism pathogenic to man. Its accomplishment will mark an era in sanitation.[15]

In 1920, Gorgas and Carter were co-authors of a paper that beamed optimism: "The brilliant work of Noguchi in discovering the organism causing yellow fever [*Leptospira icteroides*] already is having some effect on the control of the disease."[16]

Such optimism was disrupted by news that yellow fever or something like it was present in an area along the west coast of West Africa (or the western coast of Central Africa). The disease had previously been suspected in this area long known by Europeans as the "White Man's Grave."[17] The Rockefeller Foundation responded by sending a Yellow Fever Commission to the West Coast of Africa in 1920, with Gorgas in charge. Gorgas suffered a stroke en route and was taken to London, where he died at age 66. The expedition failed. Still, the Rockefeller authorities remained convinced that yellow fever could not be eradicated "until we have definitely demonstrated that this disease exists in West Africa by actual isolation of the leptospira icteroides, and until we have located the areas where it is endemic, and have further light concerning the breeding habits of the one or several factors of its transmission."[18] They accepted Noguchi's *Leptospira icteroides* as the causative agent. But was *Aedes aegypti* the only insect vector? In West Africa, unlike in the Americas, there were many closely-related mosquitoes. Was it possible that these, too, could transmit the disease?

The first Rockefeller investigator to die of yellow fever while studying the disease was Dr. Howard B. Cross, 33, a graduate of the Johns Hopkins University School of Medicine. Cross succumbed on December 26, 1921 during his assignment at Tuxtepec, Mexico. Mexico gave him the honors of a military hero, and the public health laboratory at Vera Cruz was later named for him.

The West African Yellow Fever Commission

Despite these setbacks, the Rockefeller Foundation pressed forward in 1925 with the the organization of a new West African Yellow Fever Commission. Its specific purposes were

> (1) to learn the characteristics and epidemiology of the disease in West Africa and its relationship to the fever of the Western Hemisphere; (2) to attempt the isolation of the organism which causes the disease; (3) to discover the method of transmission; and (4) to identify those areas in which the disease is continually present.[19]

The foundation chose to concentrate on southwestern Nigeria—especially the port city of Lagos and the cities and towns just to the north of it. This move was deemed "equivalent to bearding the lion in its den, for Africa is thought to be the original home of yellow fever."[20]

Henry Beeuwkes, a 43-year-old retired Army colonel, was chosen to head the new commission. Beeuwkes had no background in yellow fever, nor was he a distinguished scientist. However, he was known to be an able administrator and was fluent in French, German, and

Dutch, all of which might be useful. A Johns Hopkins medical graduate, he had rendered personal service to General John J. Pershing during the Great War. He then served on a mission to Armenia and as medical director of the American Relief Administration in Russia. Beeuwkes prepared for his task by studying yellow fever in Brazil, Guatemala, and El Salvador. In June 1925, he arrived at Lagos.[21]

The commission promptly began field surveys, for "if yellow fever is endemic on the West Coast, it must be continually occurring, probably in a mild form among the native children."[22] The Rockefeller Foundation also established a research facility on a seven and one-half acre campus located in the suburb of Yaba, five miles north of Lagos. Six buildings pre-fabricated by the Asbestos Company of Philadelphia were erected on concrete pillars. These included an office, a laboratory, an animal house, two dormitories, and a staff house. A tennis court was laid out for recreation. As the foundation noted in its annual report:

> Here live and work expert field directors, clinicians, laboratory men, assistants, and servants. This is the headquarters of the Yellow Fever Commission of the International Health Board of the Rockefeller Foundation.[23]

By the end of 1925, Beeuwkes had eight Caucasians on his staff and 54 native Nigerians, of whom 43 were at the Lagos headquarters and 11 were employed as field investigators in Ibadan, Accra, and elsewhere.[24] Beeuwkes also made arrangements to collaborate with British investigators at Accra, Gold Coast, and with French scientists at Dakar, the capital of French Equatorial Africa. Optimism ran high. For 1925, only three cases of yellow fever had been reported from the Americas. Wilbur A. Sawyer later recalled that it "seemed that complete extermination of yellow fever from the Americas and perhaps from the world was practicable and almost in sight."[25] Still—what about West Africa?

During 1926 and 1927, the researchers designed studies mainly to isolate Noguchi's spirochete, *Leptospira icteroides*, from suspected cases. They could not find it. Careful study of 67 cases suggested that

Leptospira icteroides had little if anything to do with yellow fever in West Africa. However, it was also difficult to find cases of yellow fever. The cases were widely scattered, except when epidemics occurred. Locating and examining patients early in the course of their illness was no easy matter.

Beeuwkes gave top priority to developing an animal model of yellow fever, since such a model would make isolation of the causative agent relatively straightforward. Earlier workers had tried without success. The Rockefeller investigators injected blood from patients with suspected yellow fever into various animals native to Nigeria, including monkeys. Nothing happened. Beeuwkes reasoned that the native animals might have developed resistance to yellow fever through evolution. He therefore "canvassed the animal market in New York, and in April proceeded to the Hagenbeck establishment in Hamburg."[26] Beeuwkes obtained Indian crown and rhesus monkeys from the Carl Hagenbeck firm and chimpanzees from Sierra Leone. Beeuwkes also saw the need for greater scientific expertise. He sought the help of Dr. Adrian Stokes, a pathologist at Guy's Hospital in London who had brilliantly studied typhus and cholera in the trenches during the Great War. Stokes, who was descended from a famous Dublin medical family, was granted a six month leave of absence by his employer and arrived in West Africa on May 25, 1927. The first shipment of imported animals had arrived the previous day. Everything was now in place. All that was needed was a case of yellow fever.

Stokes, Noguchi, and Young

They did not have to wait. An epidemic of yellow fever struck the town of Larteh, 32 miles northeast of Accra on the Gold Coast. On June 30, 1927, Dr. A. F. Mahaffy drew two teaspoons of blood from a 28-year-old African man named Asibi, who on the previous day had developed headache and fever. Mahaffy injected the blood into two guinea pigs, a marmoset, and a rhesus monkey designated rhesus 253-A. The guinea pigs and marmoset showed no ill effect, but rhesus 253-A developed fever on July 4 and "was found moribund and in collapse the following morning." The autopsy confirmed yellow fever and injection of that monkey's blood into a second monkey similarly caused fatal yellow fever. The virus obtained from Asibi

> was during the following months carried from monkey to monkey by inoculations of blood and serum in numerous experiments. Approximately thirty animals were inoculated in this way with fatal outcome in all instances except one; rhesus 353 developed fever but recovered.[27]

By these experiments, Stokes and his colleagues—Johannes Bauer and Paul Hudson—had proved what the Reed Commission had suggested: yellow fever is caused by a filtrable virus. It could be transmitted from human to monkey and from monkey to monkey by blood obtained early during the illness. Moreover, *Aedes aegypti* mosquitoes, once infected after feeding on infected monkeys, remained infective for other monkeys for the remainder of their lives which could be up to three months. An infected mosquito could cause fatal yellow fever with a single bite. The experiments also showed that one-tenth of a milliliter of serum obtained from a patient who had recovered from yellow fever would protect a monkey from the deadly virus if given to the monkey just before it was exposed. The susceptibility of rhesus monkeys to yellow fever was a breakthrough discovery.

The celebrating was short-lived. On September 15, 1927, Adrian Stokes became acutely ill. He was taken to the European Hospital in Lagos. Scientist to the end, he asked that his blood be drawn for inoculation into monkeys and that mosquitoes be allowed to feed on him. His only request was that a complete autopsy be carried out should he die. The autopsy confirmed yellow fever. Although there was no history of mosquito bite, all evidence indicated that "he contracted the disease while working with infected material in the Lagos laboratory."[28]

Stokes was not the only casualty. The day that Stokes became ill, Beeuwkes received notice that Noguchi himself would "shortly visit West Africa for the purpose of making investigations." Word had spread from West Africa: Rockefeller researchers had not found

Noguchi's spirochete but had found a virus instead. Sensing his reputation to be at stake, Noguchi wanted to carry out his own experiments. Beewukes was told to make adequate laboratory facilities and housing available to Noguchi at Accra. The government of the Gold Coast turned over to him a large laboratory, several smaller rooms, and "the major portion of the animal houses" of the Medical Research Institute at Accra for his use. In his report for the year, Beeuwkes wrote: "We feel extremely fortunate in having Dr. Noguchi with us, and we trust that his studies will bring to light much additional information concerning the virus of West African yellow fever."

Noguchi worked in secrecy and exactly what he learned has never been entirely clear. By May 1928, he had nearly finished his work and decided to visit the Rockefeller group at Yaba. While returning to Accra, he became acutely ill. He died two days later. Dr. W.A. Young, the director of the Medical Research Institute at Accra, performed the autopsy and confirmed the diagnosis of yellow fever. Five days later, Young became ill. He died on May 30 at age 39 of yellow fever, presumably contracted from Noguchi's infected blood. There were now four deaths.

High Hopes

Although the cost was high, the researchers had learned much about yellow fever within a short time. And it seemed likely that they could develop a vaccine. Meanwhile, the Rockefeller investigators in West Africa saw that their ability to cause experimental yellow fever in rhesus monkeys held at least four implications.

First, they could study the disease without human volunteers. They found that it took nine to 12 days for a mosquito, having bitten an infected monkey, to be infectious for a second monkey.[29] They could answer other questions about transmission. Stokes was not known to have been bitten by an infected mosquito. Would blood from an acutely ill monkey cause yellow fever in another monkey if rubbed onto the unbroken skin? It did. Yellow fever was more highly infectious than had been previously thought.[30]

Second, they could study the pathology in animals. Autopsies of infected monkeys confirmed not only the extensive damage to the liver but also widespread hemorrhage in numerous organs. Old clinical observations, including the sinister "black vomit" caused by gastrointestinal bleeding, were confirmed. They found that the yellow fever virus causes "fatty degeneration . . . in the muscle fibers of the heart."[31]

Third, they could determine from a blood sample whether a person had previously experienced yellow fever. The method was to inject the person's serum into a monkey, then inject the monkey with a dose of yellow fever virus. If the monkey survived, the patient's serum must have contained antibodies as a result of past infection. This technique, called the "protection test," was standardized by using two monkeys simultaneously. They could now determine whether mild cases and even asymptomatic cases occurred.

Last, they could determine in the laboratory which species of mosquitoes could transmit the disease by allowing mosquitoes to feed on previously-infected monkeys and then allowing the mosquitoes to feed on uninfected monkeys. Johannes Bauer showed that yellow fever could be transmitted under these experimental conditions by several mosquitoes other than *Aedes aegypti*.[32] This observation threatened to undermine the Rockefeller Foundation's basic premise that yellow fever could be permanently eradicated, since, unlike *Aedes aegypti*, these mosquitoes did not confine themselves to easily-reached environments. The fourth annual report of the West African Yellow Fever Commission noted that the

> importance of this discovery in relation to yellow fever control both in West Africa and the Americas can scarcely be overestimated. Two of these mosquitoes—the *A. luteocephalus* and *A. apicoannulatus*—are tree breeding species quite closely similar to *Aedes aegypti* in appearance and bionomics, and the fact that they are able to transmit the disease is not surprising, neither would their elimination from controlled areas offer particular difficulty. However, the positive results with *Eretmapoditis chrysogaster*, the third proved vector and a mosquito of an en-

tirely different genus, justifies the apprehension that other species impossible to control might also be capable of transmitting
the disease, and render the eradication of yellow fever from West
Africa impracticable.[33]

But the researchers were hardly ready to give up their work. Demonstration of the viral etiology of yellow fever and development of an
animal model prompted the International Health Division of the
Rockefeller Foundation to establish its own laboratory in New York,
under the direction of Dr. Wilbur A. Sawyer. Under Sawyer's
supervision, the laboratory would develop an extremely effective
vaccine using the strain of yellow fever virus originally isolated from
Asibi in West Africa. In the meantime, numerous unanswered and
partially answered questions in West Africa became the concerns of
a new commission member, Theodore Brevard Hayne.

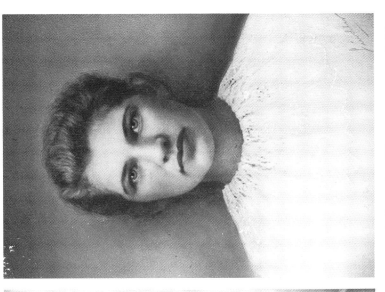

Fannie Douglass Thorn as a young bride

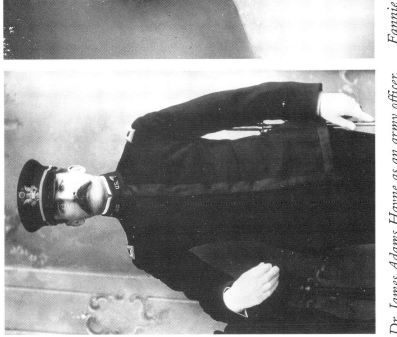

Dr. James Adams Hayne as an army officer, Spanish American War (courtesy of National Library of Medicine)

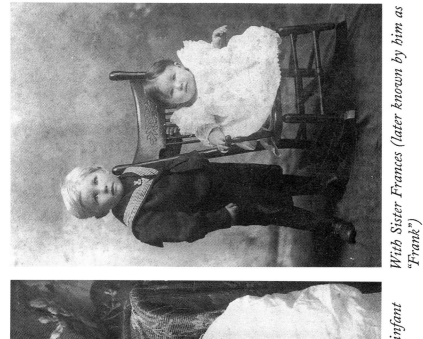

With Sister Frances (later known by him as "Frank")

Theodore Brevard Hayne as an infant

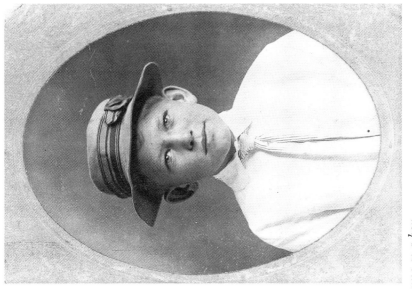

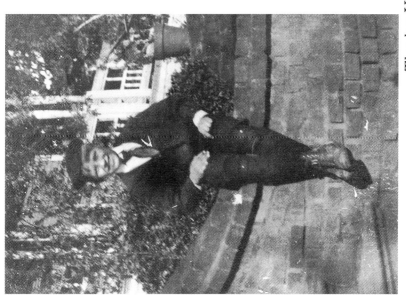

Theodore Hayne as a boy

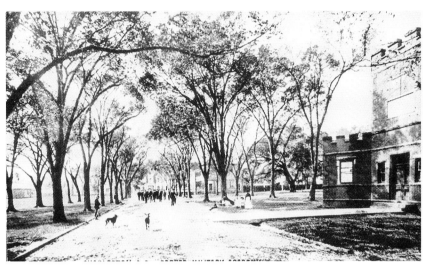

Campus and barracks of Porter Military Academy, Charleston, S.C., circa 1910–1912

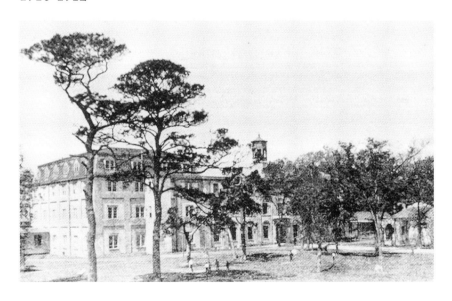

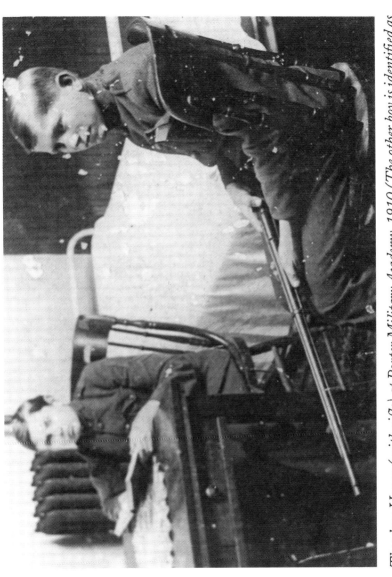

Theodore Hayne (with rifle) at Porter Military Academy, 1910 (The other boy is identified as Bryan Flemming.)

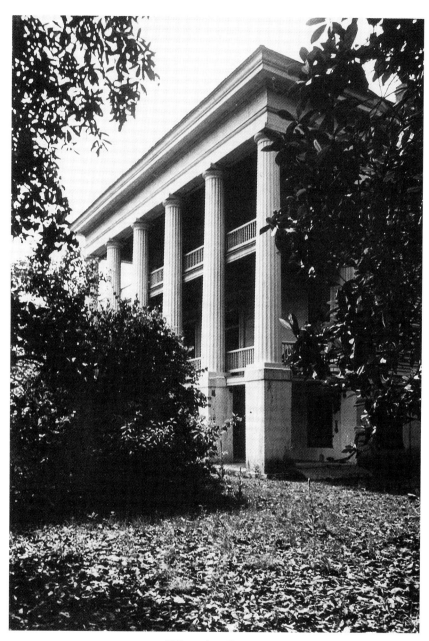

Wavering Place

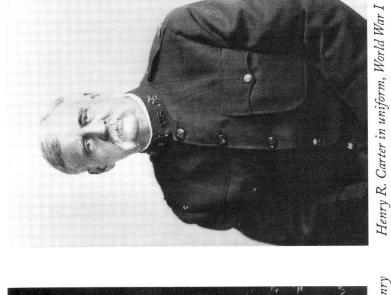

Henry R. Carter in uniform, World War I

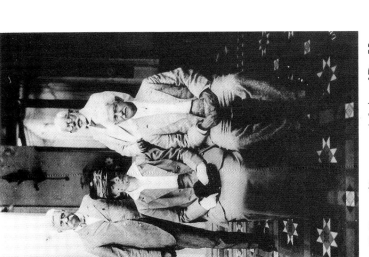

William C. Gorgas (front row, right) and Dr. Henry R. Carter (back row, left), Panama, circa 1907. Others are Mrs. Gorgas and Dr. Juan Guiteras. (courtesy National Library of Medicine)

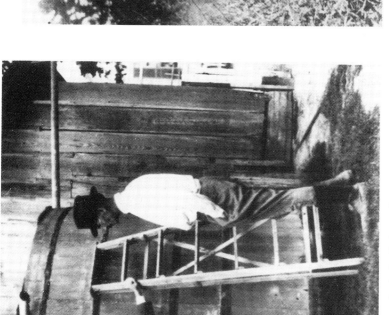
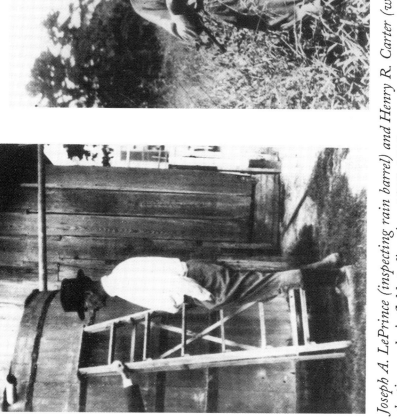

Joseph A. LePrince (inspecting rain barrel) and Henry R. Carter (with mosquito trap) conducting malaria field studies, circa 1915–1918

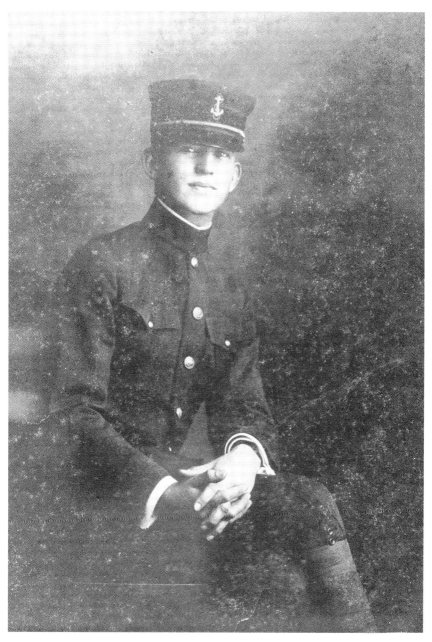

Hayne as a student at the Naval Aviation School, Seattle, Washington, in 1918

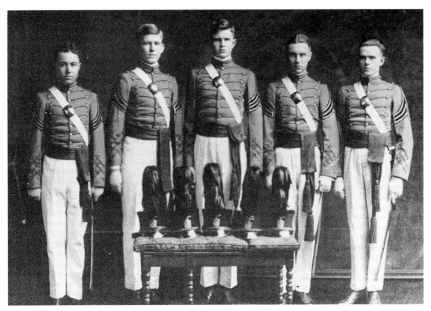

Men of Company C (Hayne is second from left). Below: The Calliopian Literary Society (Hayne is eighth from right). (Both courtesy of The Citadel Archives, Charleston, South Carolina, from The Sphinx, *1920)*

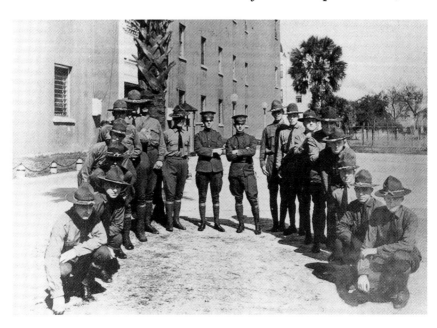

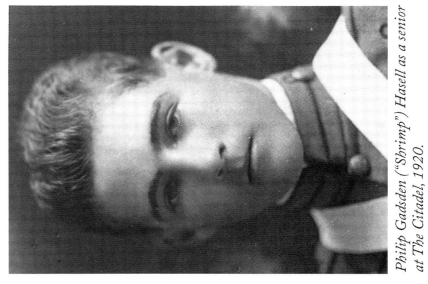

Philip Gadsden ("Shrimp") Hasell as a senior at The Citadel, 1920.

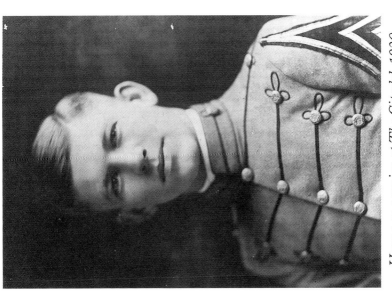

Hayne as a senior at The Citadel, 1920

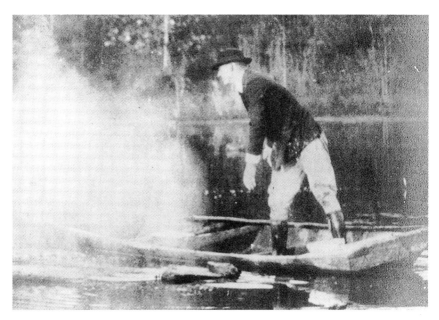

Hayne throwing from a flat-bottomed boat a sackful of Paris green (cloud at left), the mosquito larvicide he discovered with Marshall A. Barber

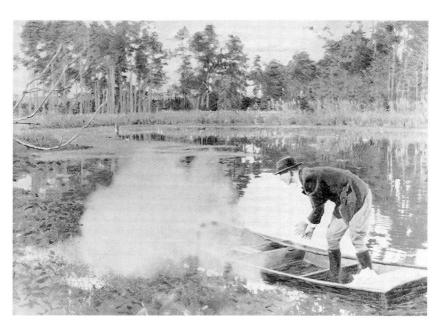

A touched-up photograph of the same scene that hung in the parlor at Wavering Place for many years

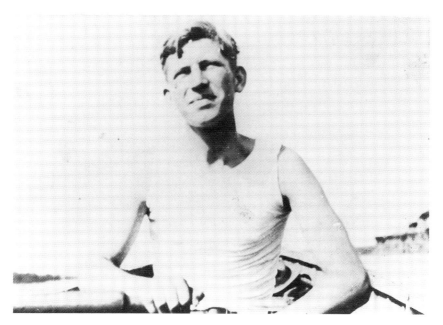

Hayne captioned this photograph "Theodore B. Hayne at work," date and location unknown

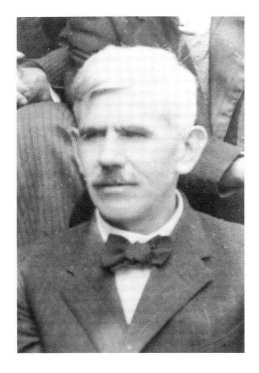

Marshall A. Barber in later life (courtesy of the University of Kansas Archives)

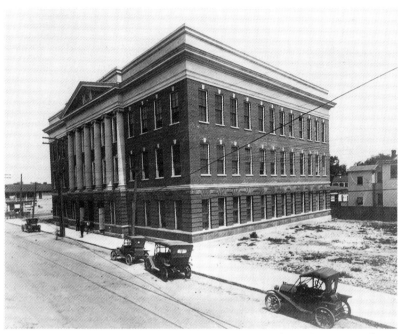

The Medical College of the State of South Carolina, circa 1914 (courtesy of the Waring Historical Library).

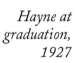

Hayne at graduation, 1927

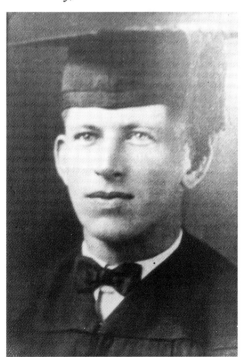

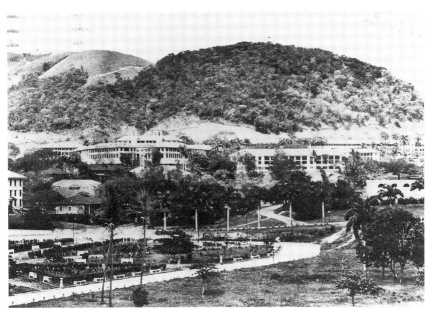

Gorgas Hospital (Ancon Hospital) with Ancon Hill in the background, Ancon, Canal Zone, circa 1928

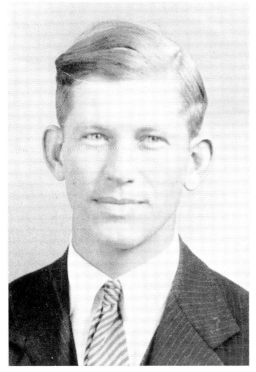

Hayne as a young man

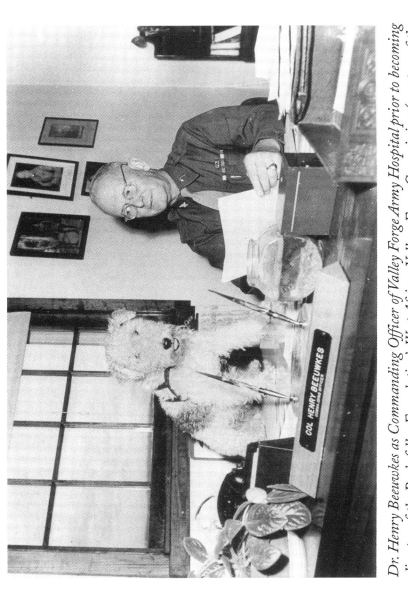

Dr. Henry Beeuwkes as Commanding Officer of Valley Forge Army Hospital prior to becoming director of the Rockefeller Foundation's West African Yellow Fever Commission (courtesy of the National Library of Medicine)

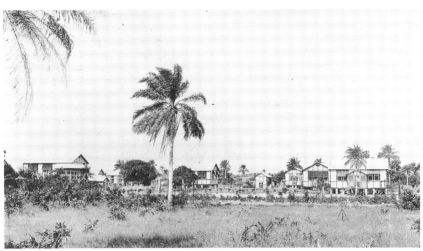

Overview of the Rockefeller Foundation's compound at Yaba, near Lagos, Nigeria (above); two laboratory buildings and an animal house, background (below) (courtesy of the Rockefeller Archive Center)

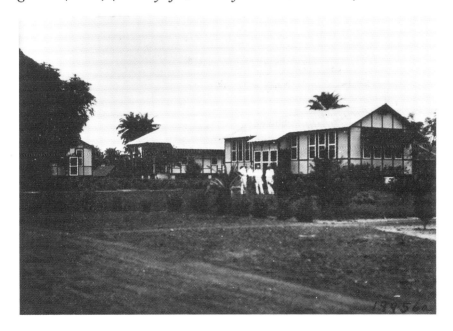

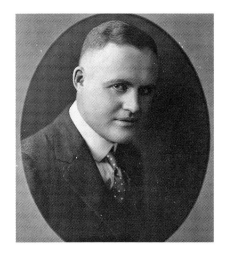
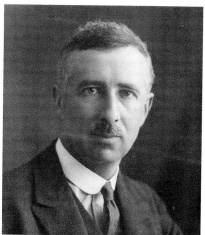
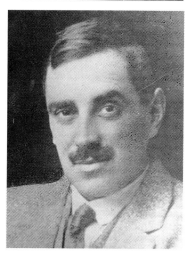

*The Rockefeller Foundation
investigators who died of yellow
fever before Hayne (clockwise from
upper left):*

*Howard B. Cross (1888–1921),
Adrian Stokes (1887–1927),
William A. Young (1889–1927),
Hideyo Noguchi (1876–1928),
and Paul A. Lewis (1879–1929)*

(courtesy of Rockefeller Archive Center)

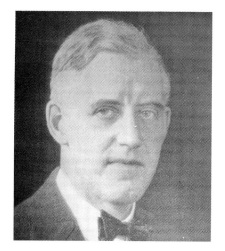
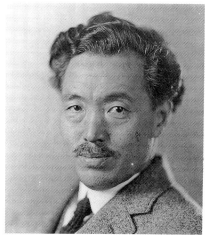

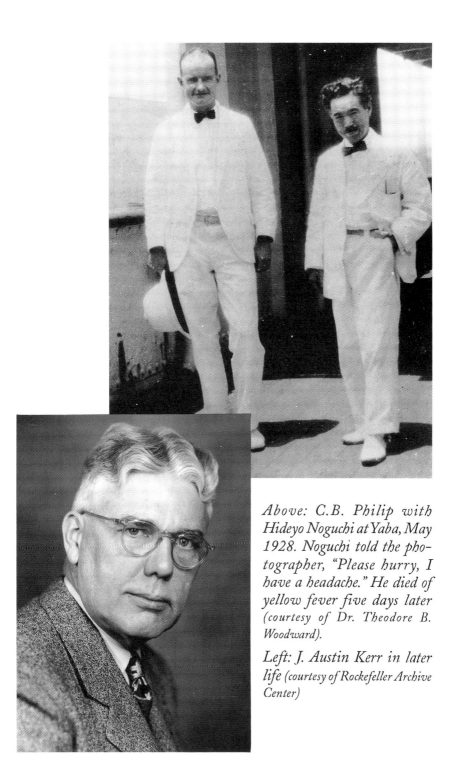

Above: C.B. Philip with Hideyo Noguchi at Yaba, May 1928. Noguchi told the photographer, "Please hurry, I have a headache." He died of yellow fever five days later (courtesy of Dr. Theodore B. Woodward).

Left: J. Austin Kerr in later life (courtesy of Rockefeller Archive Center)

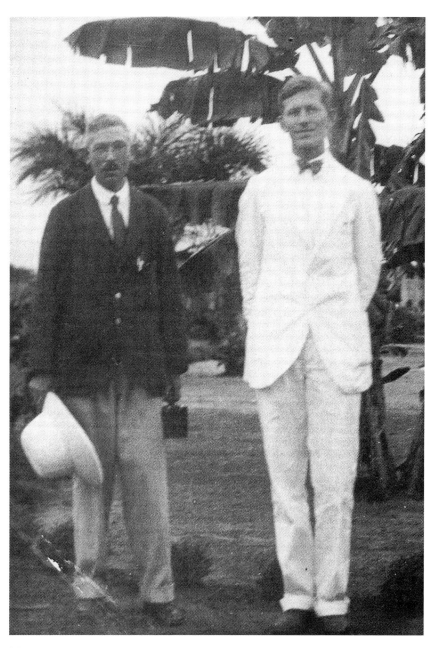

Hayne in Nigeria with a Mr. Wright—probably Ruthven Alexanderson Wright, the Anglican priest who later held a memorial service for Hayne

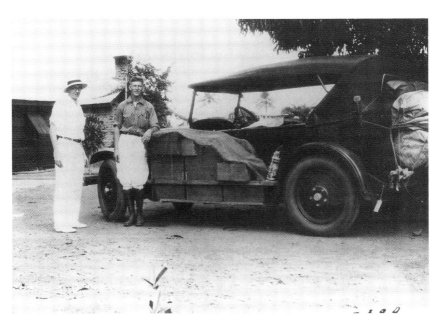

Hayne preparing for field surveillance of yellow fever cases in a specially-equipped Dodge touring car. Changing a tire somewhere in Nigeria

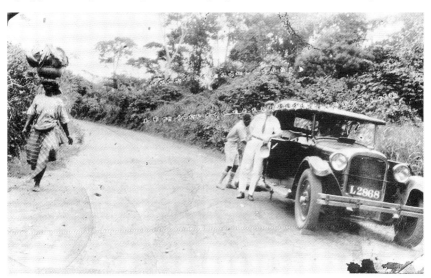

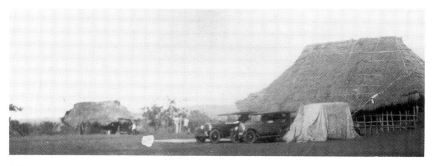

The rest house at Fugor, with Dodge touring cars used for field surveillance of yellow fever

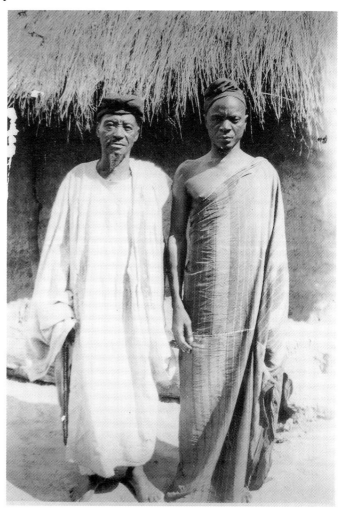

Nigerians photographed by Hayne

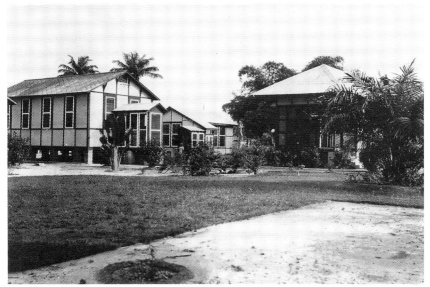

Laboratory building at Yaba (above left). Below: triple–door entry system designed to prevent mosquitoes infected with the yellow fever virus from escaping (courtesy of Rockefeller Archive Center)

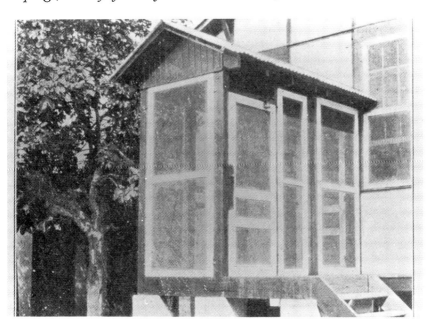

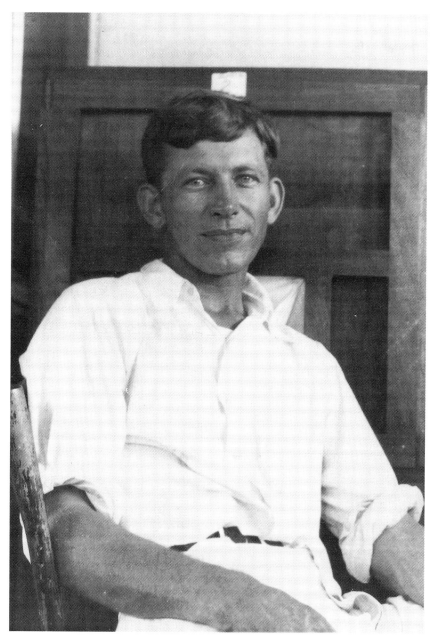

Hayne in the laboratory at Yaba, November 1929, photographed by his friend, Vladimir Glasounoff

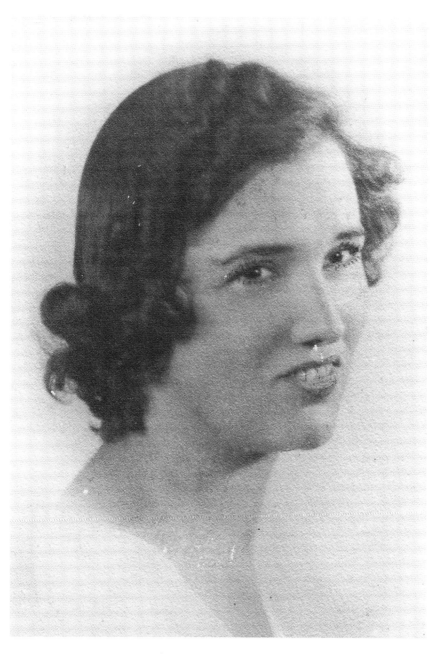

Anne Roselle Hundley

State Board of Health
of South Carolina

Columbia, S. C.

On July 5, 1930, Fannie Hayne wrote her son that "I feel so anxious about your health staying so long in the tropics." That same day, Hayne developed symptoms of yellow fever.

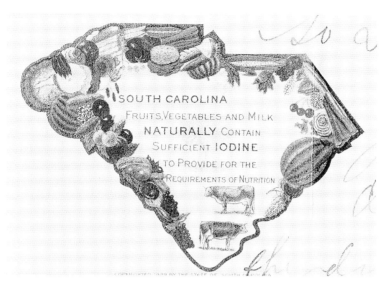

Detail of advertisement for South Carolina farm products that Adams Hayne had placed on the State Board of Health stationery on the belief that naturally-occurring iodine was superior to the pure mineral

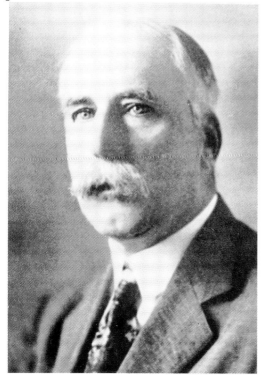

James Adams Hayne in later life

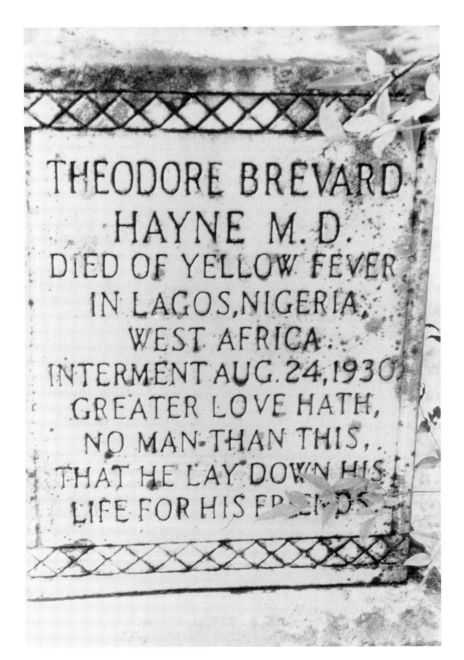

Inscription on Hayne's tombstone, St. John's Episcopal Church, Congaree, S.C.

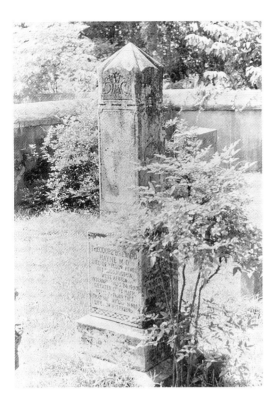

*Hayne's tombstone;
below, marker of
Theodore and Roselle
Hayne's stillborn
child, Theodora*

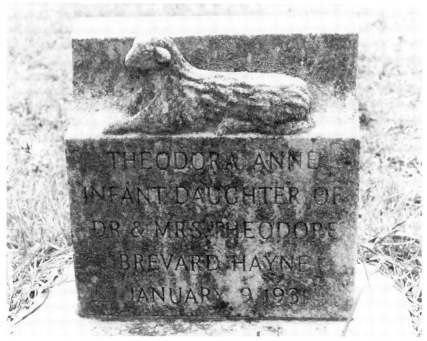

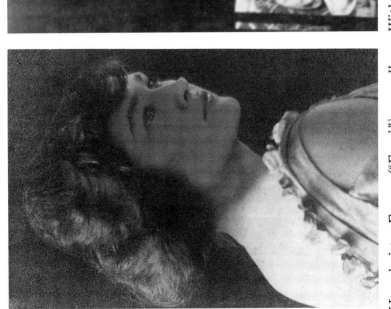

With her first child, Philip Gadsden Hasell, Jr. ("Toli" in Hayne's letters)

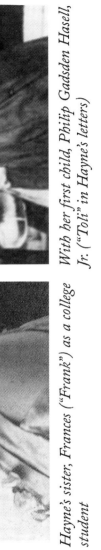

Hayne's sister, Frances ("Frank") as a college student

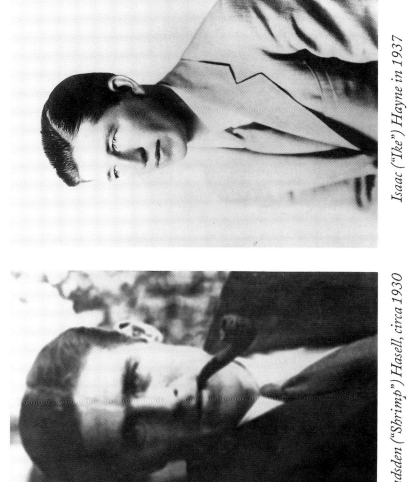

Philip Gadsden ("Shrimp") Hasell, circa 1930

Isaac ("Ike") Hayne in 1937

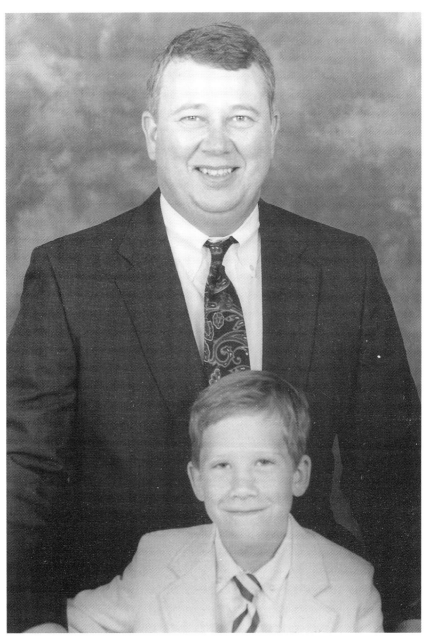

Theodore Brevard Hayne, IV, and his son, Theodore Brevard Hayne, V, in 1995

4

"A Most Satisfactory Man"

On July 4, 1928, Theodore Hayne joined the Rockefeller Foundation's International Health Division at a salary of $291.67 per month ($3500 per year), much of which he used to re-pay Laura Carter the $2200 she and her father had loaned him for medical school. Miss Carter conveyed her gratitude to Frederick F. Russell, director of the International Health Division:

> I hope that Theodore is not making these monthly payments larger than is convenient for him, for it would have been a privi-lege to help such a man get a start under any conditions. I must admit, however, that the money is a God-send at present. . . . It is almost a miracle then to have these repayments start at this particular time and I am most grateful, not only to Theodore for being so generous in the amount of his salary assigned for this purpose, but to yourself for making the present system of repayment possible.[1]

On July 6, Hayne reported to New York and was found on physical examination to be "erect, well developed and nourished," slightly over six feet tall and weighing 160 pounds, with an "even temperament," and in excellent health. The next day, he left by steamship for Liverpool, and from Liverpool he sailed for Lagos. On August 2, he reported for duty to Henry Beeuwkes at the headquarters of the West African Yellow Fever Commission at Yaba.

Life at Yaba

The staff at Yaba consisted of 21 Caucasians and 102 black Africans, of whom 31 were laboratory and office workers, 31 were stewards, and the remainder artisans, laborers, chauffeurs, and scouts. A new building had just been constructed for the animal work with infected mosquitoes. It was "small, carefully screened, and light, and if by chance a mosquito should gain entrance, it would be much more readily detected and caught than in the larger and darker main laboratory."[2]

Hayne found at Yaba a mix of veteran researchers and eager contemporaries. He soon became friends with two of the younger men: Cornelius B. (Neil) Philip and Henry William Kumm. Philip, 28, was a native of Colorado who was working toward a doctorate in entomology at the University of Nebraska. Kumm, 27, had been born in Germany of missionary parents, had braved U-boats to immigrate to the United States in 1915, and had just completed a doctorate in public health at Johns Hopkins, his medical alma mater. Both men had left their wives behind because of the dangers of yellow fever work at Yaba.

Hayne hoped that some of his family might visit him in West Africa, but his description of Lagos was less than enticing:

> It isn't quite a healthy or attractive place when you leave the water front. There are about 14 deaths a week from bubonic plague alone. . . . The quarantine is rather strict so that none of the island towns have that one dread disease. Many however are not so fortunate as regards Yellow Fever. Ife where Dr. Walcott was working has a lot. Auchi had a few. Ibadan a town of about a quarter of a million people had quite an epidemic last year.[3]

Similarly, he wrote "Shrimp" Hasell:

> The wilds here are not as wild as writers would have one believe. Disease however is very prevalent. Bubonic plague is killing lots of people every week in spite of the quarantine and strenuous efforts of the health department to stamp it out. There are more deaths per week this year than last year at the same

time in spite of the supposedly active deratting gangs that work in the town. Fortunately no cases have been found here at Yaba. You understand that our compound or set of buildings is about five miles outside the main town. Lagos itself is an Island. There have been reported a few cases in Euba Metta a part of the mainland but thus far none in the houses near us. Our buildings are very clean and well screened and the grounds are remarkably well kept. I shall try to send some pictures of the place and some good ones are taken but you can see in the last annual report of the Rockefeller Foundation what the place is beginning to look like. A couple of weeks ago we had a man in the hospital at Lagos with black water fever. He lives in Lagos and has not been out into the interior often. Almost everyone on the compound has had his go at the Flu recently. I am about the only one who has escaped. I had a bad cold last week which made [me] feel rather rotten but am all right now and am as usual in good health.[4]

Although the health situation was worrisome, there were compensating attractions. The staff at Yaba had an international flavor. A young Russian, Vladimir Glasounoff, would become a close friend. There were many English, to Hayne's amusement: "At first I didn't like my afternoon tea but am getting really English and look forward to it about four in the afternoon while working in the laboratory."[5] He wrote his sister Lillah that the

English are cuckoo about going out in the sun without sun helmets. I was warned several times on the way coming down but didn't mind that but here it's almost an insult to come to town with a Panama hat and if seen out in the sun without a hat someone will call madly to get in the shade and put on a helmet. After a year in Panama where a pith helmet and [?] down the spine were unknown it seems ridiculous. I think most of the sunstrokes here are due to drinking too much alcohol and then working in the sun. All the peripheral blood vessels are dilated permitting the heat to raise the body heat much above normal. Most of the English men Ive met here drink whiskey in the evenings as if it were water. It doesnt wonder why a mans life in tropics is shortened. Ive become an almost teetotaler. None of the men of our compound at Y[aba] drink much.[6]

Likewise, he wrote "Shrimp" Hasell:

These English people have many peculiar ideas. The first that one notices is that they have a terrible fear of the sun and wont ever go outside of the house even on a cloudy day without wearing a pith helmet. They are so absorbed in the idea that they criticize the several of us at the compound here when we are seen out in the ordinary straw hat or often none at all. The other erroneous idea is that screening of the houses prevents the breeze and makes them unbearably hot. Practically none of their houses are screened. They sit about in the evening at drinks and wear soft leather boots to prevent the mosquitoes from biting their legs but fight them off their faces and arms. They seldom work after 4 in the afternoon. Go for golf or tennis at that time and collect at six in groups at various houses for drinks and small chop (hors de oeurves) and then have dinner about 9 P.M. Ive been to a couple of the dance[s] here but they are not so good. The music is not particularly good and the dancers are little better.[7]

He confided to Hasell that he was having difficulty saving money, in part because of "buying some of the native handiwork from the Hausa men that frequent the compound." He also bought a tennis racket and some golf clubs:

It seems part of the existence out here to go to the golf course every Sunday morning at seven A.M. Im getting used to it now but find that Im no better golfer than the day I started. The game certainly requires more skill than I supposed. The tennis is not so much for me as I play such a rotten game that I can find no one who wants to play.[8]

Hayne spent most of his first four months at Yaba training for field surveillance. On August 29, Beeuwkes wrote Frederick F. Russell that

Drs. Hayne and Kumm impress me most favorably but they will require some months of training under supervision before they can be expected to carry on independently in the field. . . . Dr. Hayne is orienting himself, assisting Dr. [Oscar] Klotz in dissecting mosquitoes, and helping me in attempting to work out more satisfactory means for field transport. I contemplate sending him to Ogbomosho within a few weeks, provided some emergency does not require him elsewhere.[9]

For his part, Hayne was "rather anxious to get started work upcountry."[10] Henry Beeuwkes fully supported this desire for action. On November 1, Beeuwkes praised him even further to Russell:

Doctor Hayne is one of the most satisfactory men we have had in West Africa. He has a wonderfully attractive personality and it is a pleasure to have him about the place. At the same time he is an indefatigable worker; has a good mind and readily adapts himself to local conditions. His experience in the field and practical knowledge concerning malaria and entomology are proving valuable to us. He brought over a few simple tools with him, with which he repairs automobiles, clocks, watches, or anything else that happens to break or get out of order. He is still a little weak along literary lines such as preparation of reports, but will gradually overcome this. In any case it is better to do things well than write beautifully about relatively poor work. To my mind, too much is being written at the present time especially along medical and research lines. . . . Men of the type mentioned are far more valuable to us than the thoroughbred type of highly-trained, breast-fed, ultra-specialist, who are absorbed in academic[s] and little interested in practical problems.[11]

Jack of All Trades

On November 30, 1928, Hayne began to look for cases of yellow fever in the Ibadan district of southwestern Nigeria. Ibadan was a city of a quarter of a million people "located on hills and ridges" among which coursed the many branches of two large streams, the

Kudeti and the Ogumpo. The streams were loaded with *Pistia*, duckweed, and mosquitoes. During the rainy season, the Kudeti and Ogumpo swelled into swamps up to one-half mile in width. Marshall Barber later wrote that the "construction of houses . . . seemed to favor the comfort of the mosquito rather than that of man."[12] Near Ibadan were four cities of about 100,000 population each and numerous smaller cities and towns. The experts at the Rockefeller Foundation had theorized that if yellow fever were indeed endemic in West Africa, this would be the best place to find it.[13]

And finding yellow fever was extremely important to the Rockefeller Foundation project. As Henry Beeuwkes had grasped in 1925:

> A study of this entire area [the Ibadan district] is of vital importance for it will be necessary to clearly and definitely establish the presence of yellow fever in endemic form before we would be justified in suggesting or attempting to carry out the widespread, difficult, and expensive control campaigns that would be required to purge it of the disease.[14]

Yet it had also been predicted that field surveillance in this region would be quite frustrating. For 1926, the Rockefeller Foundation's *Annual Report* noted:

> The vastness of the area, the primitive conditions of travel, the suspicions and the superstitious traits of the population, the lack of trained personnel, the absence of centralized control, the high costs to colonial administrations will offer serious if not insuperable obstacles.[15]

Likewise the 1927 *Annual Report* acknowledged that numerous

> difficulties are met with in investigating native outbreaks. The natives run away and hide their sick when the European doctors come into town. Great tact and patience are required to gain their confidence sufficiently so that they will permit examinations to be made.[16]

Between November 30, 1929 and September 23, 1930, Hayne made 14 round trips between Ibadan and Yaba but spent all but 49 days in Ibadan and its surrounding area. The work was fraught with frustrations, as had been predicted.

The surveillance system was based on the use of trained African scouts, of whom there were three in January 1929 and eight by the end of the year. The scouts looked for people with fever or other signs of illness in Ibadan and in the surrounding cities and towns: Oyo, Abeokuta, and Ijebu-Ode. Each day, they visited housing compounds, took preliminary histories from sick persons, recorded temperatures and pulse rates, examined urine specimens, made blood smears, and prepared reports for the medical officer. The scouts were to telegram the medical officer if there was reason to suspect yellow fever. The physician would then drive out to examine the patient and make an investigation.

There were many obstacles. Most of the people received medical care largely from witch doctors known as "ju ju" men. "Ju ju pots" filled with objects intended to satisfy spirits stood before many of the houses. The pots also filled with rainwater, providing ideal habitats for mosquito larvae. The Rockefeller Foundation experts had observed that the cities "are under native administration, there are only a few small hospitals, and dispensaries, and trained medical personnel are limited to one or two Government doctors stationed in some of the towns, and a few medical missionaries."[17] Vital statistics were virtually nonexistent. The custom of burying the dead inside the houses or compounds made it even more difficult to recognize the presence of an epidemic. To complicate matters, the people were by and large suspicious of physicians.

Hayne began his work with customary enthusiasm. He described to his sister Lillah the preparations for a typical field expedition:

> There are three boxes on each side 20" long and 20" high with hinged tops cut to fit the shape of the side of the car. All cooking utensils, grub, laboratory supplies, and medicine are put in them. All clothes etc are . . . in back of car and bedding roll is

packed in a sort of grid luggage carrier attached to bumper on back. There is a rule at the Commission that only the regular native chauffeurs can drive but I made a kick to Dr. Beeuwkes and he permits me to make my trips upcountry without a driver. Most of them drive too poorly and take such chances that I almost pushed the floor boards out on my first trip. You know Im not usually nervous but these drivers are too much for me.[18]

Similarly, he wrote his brother Ike, who had begun medical school:

About next Wednesday I am to make a trip up country in the dodge touring [car] here to investigate some epidemic of jaundice which is not yellow fever. I have to take three monkeys, three rabbits, ten guinea pigs and several white rats and mice. Also I have a lot of different tubes of bacteriological media and must make some transfers of blood urine and feces into them. I hope that I can strike a good early case and on about the third week of his illness. The whole thing may be a washout but we want to at least make an effort to find out what the cause of the disease is before we leave that territory as its so easy to confuse it with mild yellow fever. It may be Weils disease or Ictero-hemorrhagica but the symptoms dont point that way. Dengue has been known to show jaundice as has Influenza[,] malta fever[,] relapsing fever and many other similar disease[s] and we want to try to be sure that it is not any of these. The slides for malaria were neg[ative]. Did I write you that I examined 150 blood slides from school children in the city of Abeokuta and found that 76% had estivoautumnal rings (P. falciparum) in their blood? The town seems to be a well drained one in the hills and it was rather surprising to me to get such a high percent.[19]

Hayne examined suspected malaria cases on his own initiative. He wrote "Shrimp" Hasell that

I am becoming a jack of all trades and am called on to do all sorts of work from auto work to diagnosing yellow fever cases . . . I dont know what will be my next job but hope that they will soon send me back in the bush as the time seems to pass much faster there. Probably it is because the work is so different every day and because we live a camp life. I shall have to improve my culinary art if I expect to survive for any length of time on my own cooking.[20]

He confided homesickness to his brother Ike:

> This is certainly a lonely existence here and if one is not at work doing something practically all of the time it certainly gets monotonous. There are no movies. The beach is too far away and the Lagoon is considered too dirty and unsafe to swim in. There was a rule here that no one could go out of the compound without a native driver for the commissions cars but I kicked so much that at last I am permitted to do my own driving.[21]

Christmas provided at least one opportunity for the young men at Yaba to celebrate with their peers. Henry Kumm recorded the details:

> We had a real Christmas feast in the mess-hall. Thirty-five people were present and enjoyed turkey and ice cream (with chocolate sauce) . . . everyone seemed happy and cheerful. I persuaded 3 of the younger men to go swimming with me at a nearby beach. Later that evening we went to Gordon's [Davis] room and made music. Philip, C.B. plays the saxaphone and Hayne the clarinet. The evening flew too soon.[22]

Henry Beeuwkes gave Hayne perfect ratings for the year in diplomacy, social activity (as a means of securing cooperation), promptness, economy, physical health, temperament, and habits. Hayne needed to improve his ability to prepare reports, articles, and public addresses. Confident about Hayne's promise, Beeuwkes indicated on January 3, 1929, that Hayne might become an independent investigator after having "an opportunity to study a few cases of yellow fever."[23]

But the cases were not forthcoming. On January 9, for example, Hayne carried out an autopsy on a suspected case only to find that "both kidneys showed small abscesses."[24] Unable to verify cases of yellow fever, Hayne found time to pursue other subjects such as surveying the mosquito population of Ibadan. His broader interest in tropical medicine did not escape Beeuwkes' attention:

> We received a diary from Dr. Hayne indicating that he has accomplished excellent work and has shown a great deal of initiative during the absence of Dr. Walcott. He has studied an interesting epidemic among the railway gang at Oshogbo, and has been able to identify the organism of relapsing fever in 3 cases among the 47 examined, or 6.4 per cent. Twenty-five and one-half per cent showed subtertial malarial parasites, and approximately 50 per cent eosinophilia. The cases of relapsing fever show a leukocytosis.[25]

To Hayne, these observations were at best imperfect consolation. In March 1929, he wrote that "I still havent seen a case and am very anxious to know what to do next year."[26] In July, he suggested that he had come to West Africa at the wrong time:

> I have been finding a number of jaundiced cases in Ife but cant seem to see any of them before the eighth or tenth day of their illness and then it is too late to take their blood to try to transfer the possible Y F to a monkey at Lagos. They certainly had the disease at this place before I arrived here last year. The strain of virus is going in the monkeys at the present time. There is reported some yellow fever in Monrovia but the president of the Liberian Republic doesn't seem to want any outsiders coming into his country to investigate. Apparently I have come to this part of the world at the wrong time to see this disease.[27]

This was indeed the case.

For reasons that were seldom apparent, yellow fever was always characterized by periodicity. In some years, it caused epidemics; in others, it seemed quiescent.[28] For 1929, yellow fever "was not reported from any part of the West Coast of Africa . . . with the exception of an epidemic of the disease in Liberia."[29] However, there were numerous illnesses that could resemble yellow fever. Some of them could be diagnosed, such as malaria, lobar pneumonia, liver abscess, and relapsing fever. There were two mysterious illnesses, one known among the natives as "Kukuruku disease" and the other as "kojupon" or "ponjuponju." Rockefeller authorities felt that yellow fever must "always be present somewhere in Nigeria," but that the obstacles to finding it were "practically insuperable at the present time."[30]

Hayne's bright disposition enabled him to tolerate these frustrations. He described domestic life at Ibadan to his mother:

> This house is full of pets now. The hospital cat "Maggie" has two kittens about a month old which have taken over the place. The pup that Dr Potts left never seems to get enough food. The red headed monkey that Capt Harris gave me is the most amusing one of the lot. The dog and monkey put on a good show when they play together. The monkey is usually tied to a post but is turned loose every afternoon. He climbs all about the mango trees and at present is enjoying the ripe mangos.[31]

He expressed his pleasure at "news that the road to Congaree was being made passable,"[32] and showed continued delight in cars on both sides of the Atlantic:

> Which one of the Graham paiges did Dad buy[?] I suppose that with its fourth speed there will be new records established between Congaree and Columbia. You ought to see me traveling about de luxe in my Dodge four touring car with my bedding in a rack on the back and all medical supplies[,] foods [and] cooking utensils on the side running boards in boxes. . . . The last time I drove down from Ibadan to Lagos 108 miles it took 2 hours 45 minutes. This was done in a whippet 4 touring somewhat loaded. The road is tar bound macadam for about 60 miles but the other is rough. Oshogbo is 85 miles via Ede. We made that in two hours and a half. Not bad considering the load of four people and a heavy load of boxes and bedding.[33]

His personal finances remained tenuous. Beeuwkes reported that Hayne had "been robbed or has lost his wallet containing 15 pounds" and that the loss would not be covered by the Commission's insurance policy.[34] However, the foundation trusted Hayne with its automobile purchases:

> This week I went to Lagos to see about buying a car for the commission. There was a 1928 Pontiac, Dodge 6, Whippet and Oakland 6 to pick from. I got the Dodge for 275 pounds here. It was 35 pounds cheaper than Oakland and 25 more than the Pontiac.[35]

Hayne's love of cars almost became his undoing.

A Close Call

On Saturday, May 11, 1929, Hayne was returning home from "dining with the District Officer, Mr. Palmer," in Ibadan when the headlights on his Dodge suddenly went out as he proceeded down a hill at 25 to 30 miles per hour. The road had no shoulder, and there was a four foot drop to a "very bumpy surface" below. The car left the road, travelled about 40 feet, and came to rest on its roof. The roof and windshield were demolished. When Hayne regained consciousness, he was lying beside the car. He had only a slight abrasion of the right wrist. The headlights had come back on and were pointing up the hill from which he had come.

Hayne turned off the lights and walked up hill to the bungalow of a Dr. O'Carroll. The next morning, his neck was badly swollen and there was numbness in the back of the head "following the distribution of the great occipital nerve" on the right side. He experienced "numbness and tingling in the fingers of his right hand."[36] He was taken to the European Hospital in Lagos for observation. Henry Beeuwkes visited the scene of the accident and marvelled: "How Dr. Hayne escaped being killed or seriously injured it is impossible to imagine."[37] On May 26, Beeuwkes recorded: "Dr. Hayne returned to Ibadan today. He has apparently completely recovered and states that he feels quite well and is anxious to return to duty."[38]

Although he played down his symptoms to his superiors, Hayne regretted that he had been hospitalized. On June 2, he wrote his mother:

I spent a week in Lagos getting my neck etc x-rayed. I felt sure there was nothing broken but Dr Mahaffy & Dr. Mackey were not. Well there was nothing broken in the X Ray plates. The neck is still rather stiff & painful & of course limited in movement but its getting better every day. The biggest mistake I made was allowing myself to stay in the European hospital here. Of course there could be no treatment for me & I just stayed in bed for the mosquitoes to feed on me. Naturally a lot were infected from the numerous cases of malaria treated in the hospital. I got a good case of malaria just two weeks after my stay in the hospital. Fortunately I started on 45 grains of quinine daily as soon as I noted fever so that it only lasted 24 hours. I found only a few estivoautumnal parasites all small rings and no crescents. There are none now. I kept up 30 gr a day for 3 days & am on ten now so am all right again. Of course I didnt have much energy during the week but I feel much better today.

This seems to have been my hard luck month. I know my luck will change. I havent done much real work for about three weeks now but feel like getting back now. Expect to make a trip to Ijebu Ode this afternoon.[39]

On June 19, he acknowledged the close call but was able to laugh about it:

My neck and back are much better. I drive all over the country but the muscles tire easily & there is considerable pain in neck and between shoulders in the evening. That's to be expected for I had a first class wreck and just missed getting my neck broken. I suppose I inherit a rather tough neck from Col. Isaac Hayne who was hung. A sort of evolution process.[40]

On June 27, he wrote that his neck was "a little stiff and there is some limited motion but it is steadily improving." On June 30, he appended another touch of humor:

The car that I turned over in is still in Lagos. The differential was taken from it to put in my original dodge. They are still waiting for parts to repair it. Fortunately all of the damage was covered by insurance. It has a very good engine and its only fault was the loose wire in the switch that I discovered at a rather critical time. My neck is still rather stiff and there continues a small area of anesthesia following the course of the right greater occipital nerve on the back of my head. This of course in no way incapacitates me and will probably be useful in case I have a large wife who is useful with a rolling pin.[41]

Despite the accident, cars continued to fascinate him:

No one has written me how Dads car is getting along. Nothing was said of the trip to Louisville. I wondered how it made out. Which car is this of Hams that broke up on the start? Has he purchased a new one since I left? Shrimp must certainly be getting good mileage out of his tires and good service with the car. The Fords that I have seen out here get to look rather rusty and a sort of mould grows between the layers of the wind shield but the engines run perfectly. They use more Reo speed wagons or trucks than anything else here. There is a brockway truck also that is very popular with the natives. Its made in New York I believe. The English trucks or lorries as they are called are not very popular except for government use. They are apparently much more expensive than any of our trucks. My Dodge has gone 22,000 miles and is still running well. The bearings have never been touched and it doesnt knock at all.[42]

On July 10, 1929, Hayne's transfer to the regular staff was approved by the Scientific Directors of the Rockefeller Foundation at a meeting in New York. Russell wrote Beeuwkes that Hayne "was well spoken of by a number of the men present and I am sure he will be a valuable addition to our regular staff."[43] Russell wrote Hayne: "It is a great pleasure to me to welcome you to our small group."[44] His salary remained $3500 per year plus traveling expenses and "allowance for rent, board and laundry." Beeuwkes was delighted:

His service with the Commission has been most satisfactory in every respect. He is a man of most pleasing personality and his qualifications and training will make him a valuable asset to our organization. He knows and does many things in an unusually satisfactory manner and shows constant desire to improve himself and increase his usefulness.[45]

Recovered from his accident, Hayne continued to be in a good frame of mind. He reported to his mother:

The flower garden is doing fine [in] this wet weather. There are lots of Zinnias, Marigolds, and roses in bloom. The pride of Barbadoes, single red and double salmon colored hibiscus are flowering well. There are some beautiful cannas. One gorgeous red, a pink, and various yellows with pink markings. The Crotons and other varicolored leafed shrubs are growing beyond the gardeners speed at keeping them trimmed and trained.[46]

And although he had not been able to find an active case of yellow fever, his work was nevertheless useful in determining the extent of the yellow fever problem in West Africa.

Protection Tests Show Yellow Fever to be Widespread

Hayne obtained blood samples for the "protection tests" which enabled the researchers to map out the distribution and extent of the disease—a form of disease surveillance now known as "seroepidemiology."

The blood samples that Hayne had taken in the Ibadan district and elsewhere proved to be invaluable. His letters told the story months before it was reported in the scientific literature. In April 1929, he wrote his mother:

Of 25 sera taken from native people in Ibadan between ages 20-30 ten protected monkeys from contracting yellow fever when injected. This would indicate that about 40% of the Ibadan people had probably had Y.F. in the past. I can't seem to find any cases here at present however.[47]

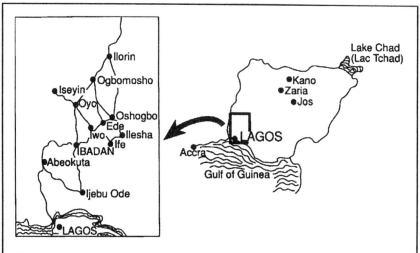

Locations of Hayne's yellow fever field surveillance in Nigeria, 1928-1929. Ibadan District is shown in the inset.

In June, he wrote:

> I'm busy keeping up with the nature scouts in Ilorin, Oshogbo, Ife, Oyo, Ijebu Ode and Ibadan. Ife is the only place that needs careful watching at present. There have been 15 cases in the last 6 weeks. All were jaundiced and at least two definitely yellow fever. Protection tests from 75 people (natives) in Ibadan gave 24 protections in monkeys. This means that a high percent of the Ibadan population is immune from Y F due to having had it sometime in the past. None of those from Jos (35) had any protective properties in their sera. This is to be expected as this town is on the plateau and free from Aedes aegypti mosquitoes.[48]

In July, he was even more encouraged:

> The protection tests of 100 people taken from the natives of Ibadan have given 32 protections in the monkeys. This means that a fair percentage of the people of this town are immune to yellow fever. This immunity has been due to having had the

disease in the past at some time. The majority must contract the disease when very young for of twenty five that were five years of age six gave positive protection to the monkeys. The lot of thirty five taken from Jos on the plateau all failed to protect the monkeys indicating that the disease had never been in that area. Those from Kano are going to show that yellow fever has not been that far north also tho these tests are not completed.[49]

These data confirmed that yellow fever was endemic in Nigeria. More specifically, yellow fever was endemic in the heavily-populated Ibadan district near the coast, where nearly two-thirds of randomly-selected people had antibodies. However, in smaller, remote inland towns such as Jos, Zaria, and Kano, the disease seemed to be virtually non-existent.[50]

Hayne attempted to take the antibody determinations one step further. Was it possible to predict, on the basis of a person's medical history, whether serum would contain antibodies against the yellow fever virus? It had been observed that "histories may be very valuable, and positive histories of yellow fever among West Africans were often correct."[51] Hayne studied the medical histories and protection test results in 76 West Africans. Beeuwkes had asked him to obtain "as accurate information as possible on the illnesses of these persons." He sent his scouts, who did not know the protection test results, to question people about their illnesses. According to Beeuwkes, "if information secured by a scout was entirely negative, he sent a second scout and the histories of the two do not always agree." When the information obtained by the scouts was confusing, Hayne would try to resolve the matter himself.

The data were promising. Of the 20 people who gave histories suggestive of yellow fever, 12 had confirmatory protection test results. Of the 56 people whose histories did not suggest yellow fever, only 14 had positive protection test results. Hence, the hypothesis that the history might predict the result seemed correct.[52] However, there were problems with the data. Beeuwkes lamented that "I am rather afraid that most of our scouts are not sufficiently reliable or intelligent to carry out work of this kind, and some of them may deliberately bring in the information they think we desire, and without any reference to the actual statements of the patients."[53]

Although it was difficult to correlate the histories with the protection test results, the data held implications. Yellow fever was a common disease in parts of West Africa. The results were summarized in the Rockefeller Foundation's annual report:

> In applying this test to a considerable number of African natives the discovery was made that a large percentage of them must at some time have had yellow fever, since even a minute quantity of their serum was sufficient to protect monkeys. As these persons frequently did not remember having had yellow fever at all, the conclusion is inescapable that they must have had it in a light form.[54]

It was further noted that the "important part played by the African native in the perpetuation of yellow fever has long been suspected. Sir Rubert Boyce, who wrote a book on yellow fever in 1911, was of the opinion that the African native is as saturated with yellow fever as he is with malaria."[55]

Back to Entomology

Hayne's ability to work with and think about mosquitoes was not wasted. In Ibadan, he collected "large numbers of mosquito larvae." He sent them to Lagos "to determine whether or not a particular species is capable of transmitting yellow fever." He sent four lots containing 16,000 larvae of a common swamp-breeding mosquito now known as *Mansonia africana*.[56] Only a small percentage of the larvae survived the trip, but these mosquitoes transmitted yellow fever in the laboratory. This mosquito commonly bred "in the water celery, or Pistia, of the sluggish ponded streams of Ibadan and other towns of the north" and was "a vicious biter of man." Hayne also collected larvae of a rock pool-breeding mosquito known as *Aedes vittatus (sugens)* from the rock holes of Abeokuta. This species could also transmit yellow fever in the laboratory. The results gave additional credence to the notion that *Aedes aegypti* was not the only vector.

Hayne kept up his interest in malaria, which was common among the Caucasians at Yaba. It was frequently acquired at the garden parties or in the unscreened houses occupied by the English. Quinine usually stood on the lunch tables; the recommended dose for prevention was six grains daily.[57] Hayne even suggested to his mother that she send blood slides from South Carolina, presumably for his amusement:

> I wish that when the folks at home get sick with malaria someone would take a blood slide thick and thin and send to me. Of course it would not be heard from in time to be of any use in treatment but it would satisfy my curiosity with regard to the diagnosis.[58]

In July 1929, he explained that he carried out his own malaria investigations during his spare time:

> Last week I examined the blood of twenty five native boy scouts that are going to England to some sort of jamboree and found that 18 or 72% had malaria parasites in their blood. It seems a shame that these boys were not cleared of parasites before going to England. It is in this way I suppose that malaria is replanted in areas that are at the present free from the disease. The largest percent that I have obtained thus far has been from a group of 66 children in school here in Ibadan. Of this number 64 had parasites in their blood. Several had filaria also. Almost all showed eosinophilia which was probably due to intestinal parasites. This examination of the various groups this way is being done entirely on my own in the spare time as the commission here is only interested in Yellow Fever and the laboratory experiments with the monkeys.[59]

Hayne also made observations about relapsing fever and schistosomiasis.

Immersed though he was in his work, Hayne was thinking about his future. In November 1928, he had written to his mother that

> I certainly would like to know what sort of work the commission might give me to do when I leave here. They often permit their men to take some course at a school or assign them to some work in the states before again sending them away to some foreign country. I suppose that I can only be patient and wait until I return to the U.S. to find out.[60]

In June 1929, he indicated that he did not especially want to return to West Africa:

> I dont know what I am to do when I get thru with my four months vacation after leaving here. I suppose that the commission will ask that I come back here and I am fairly sure that it wouldnt be best to do that. I do want to get something to do in malaria work. I dont know what the chances will be with the Commission or where they will want to send me. I am very much interested in the Gorgas Memorial Research Labortory in Panama and am anxious to find out what is to be done there. It would be of course much better to remain with the I H B if I can be given something more encouraging than looking for yellow Fever in West Africa.[61]

In July, he added:

> The I H B has given no indication as to the work that I shall be required to do after leaving here. As a matter of fact there is no absolute certainty, I suppose, that they will have need of my services.[62]

However, Hayne had two reasons to be optimistic: Marshall Barber and entomology.

Barber, Hayne's mentor from Public Health Service days, had joined the Rockefeller staff and was coming to Yaba. C.B. Philip, the entomologist at Yaba, was returning to the United States. Hayne explained the situation to his mother:

> Mr Philip the entomologist here is expecting to leave shortly after Dr Barbers arrival and I hope that it may be possible for me to go to Lagos to spend a while in the laboratories there

until the dry season starts. There doesnt seem to be any yellow fever about this time. I have lived a year here with the expectation of finding the disease the next day but thus far there have been no proved cases.[63]

Prior to Philip's scheduled departure on October 1, Hayne was placed in charge of the entomology laboratory at Yaba. On September 20, Beeuwkes wrote in his diary:

> As a large amount of entomological work remains to be done, and as Dr. Hayne is qualified to make studies of this character, especially those requiring field investigations, I have, after consulting with Dr. Barber and other members of the staff, invited Dr. Hayne to take over the work of Mr. Philip. Dr. Barber heartily approves of the move, both because he believes Dr. Hayne well qualified, and also because the latter has spent all of his time since his arrival in West Africa in search for cases of yellow fever in the Ibadan area and other points. As the results have not been stimulating, I would like him to have an opportunity to undertake more promising work.
>
> Drs. Hayne and Kumm arrived from Ibadan this evening, and Dr. Hayne has expressed great pleasure in accepting this entomological detail.[64]

In Ibadan, Kumm regretted the change: "I miss Ted Hayne here, he was such excellent company. He is very happy to be back in the lab at Yaba, doing the entomological work he likes best."[65]

This transition sealed Hayne's eventual fate. However, everyone was aware of the dangers inherent to working with the infected broods at Yaba. Philip had been bitten by an infected mosquito on at least one occasion. He had immediately injected himself with convalescent serum, which "may well have saved his life."[66] On October 3, Beeuwkes documented that he had undertaken all precautions:

> Dr. Hayne is taking over the entomological laboratory and making a thorough clean up before undertaking any other work. Some additional mosquito cages are being constructed in order

to make certain that our supply of normal insects will always be adequate. Dr. Bauer and I have gone over the entire field and technique with Dr. Hayne in order to secure proper coordination in the work, and have made certain changes with a view to assuring maximum safety to those carrying out the experiments.[67]

Hayne soon became quite busy with this work. On November 5, for example, Beeuwkes recorded: "Mosquitoes carried out in Ife were sorted out by Dr. Hayne, the procedure requiring a whole day. He finds a total of 561 female *Aedes aegypti*."[68] However, there was a problem. Mosquitoes were escaping from their cages. Beeuwkes wrote:

> Since Dr. Hayne has been carrying out the entomological work, very much larger numbers of mosquitoes had been used than previously. Dr. Hayne has noticed that a few mosquitoes apparently escaped from the individual cages which are stored in the double screened mosquito house. In carrying out work recently with the male *Stegomyia* [*Aedes aegypti*], several escaped promptly from the cages and were caught in the room. We have in the past always used a very fine wire, 20 or 24, for the individual cages, but a larger mesh (18) was used in some cages more recently made and also to replace corroded screen in some older cages. Female *Stegomyia* vary considerably in size and the males are of course smaller than the females, and pass quite readily through a 18 mesh gauze. I did not know that any of the latter was being used, but we will take steps to replace all of the large mesh with fine wire as soon as a consignment of the latter, ordered in August, arrives.
>
> In the meantime in order to protect the workers and to prevent the possibility of strains being crossed or experiments confused by the escape of mosquitoes from one cage into another, Mrs. Beeuwkes is working overtime in making sacks of muslin to cover each of our 44 individual cages. These will be used at least until the new gauze arrives and probably longer if it is found that the diminished accumulation of air does not exert a deleterious influence on the insects.[69]

On November 20, Beeuwkes wrote:

> After further discussion with Drs. Hayne and Bauer we have decided to cover the new mosquito enclosure which we are constructing with No. 26 mesh mosquito screening. We feel that this is a wise move, for though the enclosure may be uncomfortably warm at times due to the diminished circulation of air, we will eliminate all possibility of the escape of insects from the enclosure. I have accordingly requested by cable two additional rolls of this screen.[70]

Hayne wrote home of his concern:

> It has been a busy week here in the mosquito laboratory. A lot of the infected mosquitoes were escaping from one of the smaller cages in the infected room and I find that the size of screening being used is too large a mesh to prevent the small[est] of the mosquitoes from escaping. They have now been covered with gauze but it will be sometime before new screening arrives. It seems rather strange that they should have been working with mosquitoes here for about two years and were not sure of the proper size of screen to use on the cages containing the infected mosquitoes.[71]

There is no record that Hayne ever complained to Beeuwkes about this issue.

Marshall Barber, full of ideas as usual, raised the possibility that *Anopheles* mosquitoes might transmit yellow fever. It was an unlikely speculation, but would be sensational if true. On October 13, Beeuwkes recorded that Barber and Hayne would "shortly carry out an experiment to determine beyond any doubt whether it is possible or not to transmit yellow fever by the bites of the *Anopheles* mosquito."[72] Barber had been watching larvae developing in the pools and burrow-pits around Yaba, and had collected "many thousands of larvae" for this purpose. However, the *Anopheles* mosquitoes did "not bite monkeys readily," and most of them died in captivity.[73] Although Barber's suggestion was not verified, his presence at Yaba had rekindled Hayne's enthusiasm. Beeuwkes informed Frederick F. Russell in New York about his plans for Hayne and entomology:

> Referring to personnel:—As you know Mr. Philip left Lagos October 1st, and Dr. Hayne is taking over the work in the ento-mological laboratory. We are all satisfied that the move is a wise one, and Dr. Barber is enormously pleased, and is already plan-ning certain cooperative studies with him. We hope to limit the work in the entomological laboratory to more definite and con-crete problems than in the past, and more closely correlate it with the field and laboratory studies in general. This will make for greater safety and, I feel, for more definite and clean cut results than can be attained by one who is undertaking investi-gations of too many problems simultaneously. Dr. Hayne is very enthusiastic and has already expressed a desire to return to Af-rica after leave.[74]

However, Hayne was looking forward not only to working with mosquitoes and Marshall Barber but also to his marriage.

Looking Forward . . . and a Letter From Father

Despite the long separation, there is no indication that Hayne had any romantic interests other than Roselle Hundley. Early in his tour, he had written his sister Lillah that if "you managed to save any money you might come to my wedding in Paris about January 1930."[75] He also confided to "Shrimp" Hasell:

> There is only one unmarried person in this part of the world and she is engaged to some sot here that cant seem to ever stay sober long enough to get married. The girl is no ones angel and would crowd one too much on the front seat of a Ford on ac-count of her excess adipose tissue.[76]

In mid-1929, Roselle visited the Hayne family in Congaree. Hayne wrote his mother:

> I suppose that by this time Roselle has been to Congaree and

everyone has recovered from seeing such a tall girl. She said she was returning to Panama because there was nothing else to do.[77]

However, Hayne had heard little or nothing from his father. Adams Hayne was preoccupied with the economy, iodine, and pellagra. Pellagra had now been recognized to be a treatable cause of chronic debility and dementia in the Southeastern United States. Adams Hayne was supervising efforts to make Brewer's yeast available to those who needed it.[78] His preoccupation with iodine was motivated largely by economics—South Carolina's and his own. The low incidence of goiter in the state was attributed to the high iodine content of its soil. Adams Hayne promoted the high iodine content of South Carolina fruits and vegetables with the aim of helping the state's struggling farm economy, which included his own agricultural efforts at Wavering Place. Holding forth on this subject at the 44th Annual Conference of State and Provincial Health Authorities of North America, he was at his peak of notoriety and influence.[79] The eldest son complained to his mother: "James Adams should wrap his thumb and index fingers about a pen and spread a little news and cheer in a letter to me."[80] Finally, on November 5, Adams Hayne wrote to "my dear Theodore" what he called his "annual letter." The letter revealed an introspective and articulate man who cared deeply about his family and who had some reservations about the upcoming marriage.

Adams Hayne began with an account of the recent marriages of two daughters:

> Susan's marriage was a great shock to me. I looked upon her as a mere child and George seemed only an overgrown boy, and although he was all the time at the house I never had any idea that they contemplated matrimony. They seem, however, to be very happy and George is working hard for a small salary. They are comfortably situated in their own rooms and seem to be able to make both ends meet somehow or other, which is frequently not the case with much larger incomes. Mary had a beautiful wedding and everyone said that she made a lovely bride. We

hated much to give her up as she was the practical member of the family and always could be depended upon to do the thing she was asked to do. We miss her greatly when it comes to attending to the little errands that are necessary for housekeeping in the country when shopping has to be done in towns. Old Wavering looked lovely the night of the reception and many people remarked upon the beauty of the old place. I told them it looked much better by night than it did by day for the sunlight of day reveals the shabbiness of the house and furniture.

Next, he related his public recognition was more than offset by personal problems and depression:

This has been an extremely disagreeable year for me for since April I have been bedeviled by an alleged audit of my accounts. This audit instead of being an audit seems to be a general detractive study of my methods of conducting an office with a view of showing my unfitness to operate a business office. I never claimed to be a business man nor to have much idea about finances. I never could manage my own finances and I seem to have made a failure in managing other people's. The whole thing has been extremely mortifying to me and this six months of continued worry has aged me a great deal. I have lost most of the zest for living and am afflicted with what the medical writers call "tedium vitae" or burden of living. I have given eighteen years towards building up a Health Department for the State of South Carolina and have done my best under very trying circumstances at times to see that the State received the benefit of the money expended for public health. The vital statistics of the State show that this eighteen years has shown tremendous progress in the reduction of sickness and the diminution of the number of deaths in the State. Whether this is due to the efforts of the State Health Department or to many other causes I am unable to say. I miss your presence from this country greatly. I have no close associates nor intimate friends, and when I need advice have to turn to comparative strangers. I hate to write to you in this gloomy manner but I naturally feel gloomy. Perhaps it is the let-down after the excitement of Mary's wedding.

He offered some fatherly advice on his son's upcoming marriage:

> Roselle visited us and I was sorry that I saw so little of her. She has a great deal of dignity and poise and made a very favorable impression upon the family. I would consider, however, very seriously the question of marriage. If you feel that she is a person to whom you can turn and that she will stand by you whether you are right or wrong, whether you are guilty or not guilty, that she will be cheerful under the many vexatious things that will occur in the lives of all married people, that she will forget the little causes of disagreement and think only of your mutual welfare, if you love her sufficiently to be blind to such faults as all of us have and if she loves you sufficiently to be willing to put up with the many imperfections which she is certain to find in you as you are human, then you may be assured that marriage will be a success; otherwise the union of two people who are dissimilar in tastes who cannot mutually bear with each other is hard on either.

He concluded:

> Malaria is very prevalent in this State this year—more so than it has ever been. I wish we had you here to help the people of the State combat this disease. It is a shame that nothing is being done towards its prevention in a civilized State. Twenty-one people died in Orangeburg last month from malaria, which seems almost incredible. . . .
>
> You now have only three months from the date of this letter to remain in Africa, and when this reaches you only two. We are all anxious to see you and talk over your experiences on the dark continent. The life that you are leading is the life that attracted me as a young man, and I would have given anything at your age to have the experience which you are now getting. Your success is a great comfort to me and I feel that at least one mem-

ber of the family is out of the reach of the poverty entailed by the production of a product such as cotton, which does not pay for the cost of production. The farm this year cost me about $1800 and my salary and I see no hope for the farmer in South Carolina.

I am sending you under separate cover a copy of the pamphlet read by me at Washington on "Endemic Goitre and Its Relation to Iodine Content of Food." You have seen much of this in the newspapers and upon the iodine content of South Carolina vegetables is built the hopes of the farmers of South Carolina. Whether it will prove a "Castle in Spain" I cannot say but it has at least given hope, which is well-nigh extinct, to the farming population of South Carolina.[81]

This was the last known letter from father to son.

Homeward Bound

Any hope of a Paris wedding had long vanished. Hayne had no money. He wrote his mother that he also needed clothes:

I certainly will have to get home soon to get some clothes. All of mine are giving out. I ordered some from Sears and Roebuck sometime ago and got a reply recently saying that they could not send anything to Africa and advised to write a letter to the Globe Packing Company of New York who would make the order and repack the shipment for foreign export. I would have done this but I found that I would probably leave for home in December so that the clothes would not arrive before I left. There are some things sold locally but they are expensive and not nearly so good as those obtained at home.[82]

He was advanced 200 pounds in order to make purchases in Europe. Beeuwkes noted: "He will owe the Board approximately $400 when he arrives in New York and will balance this with a personal check."[83]

On December 5, Hayne left Lagos on the S.S. *Ussukama*. Although bound for England, he stopped over at Freetown, Sierra Leone, to investigate the possibility that yellow fever was active in that location. Beeuwkes and others had been apprehensive about whether the public health officials would be cooperative. Hayne proved to be an excellent ambassador for the Rockefeller Foundation. He drew blood samples from children that helped confirm that "Sierra Leone does not constitute an endemic area and that the disease has not been prevalent there at least during the last decade."[84] Later, Beeuwkes was informed about the value of Hayne's visit by Dr. MacDougall, the District Medical Director in Sierra Leone:

> We received a letter from the D.M.S., Sierra Leone, in which he states that Dr. Hayne's visit was greatly appreciated and that he had never had a more delightful guest, and that it was a genuine pleasure to have him in the house and to show him around. He asked to be allowed to extend what hospitality he can to any other member of the staff who has occasion to visit Sierra Leone.[85]

Finally, on December 15, Hayne left Sierra Leone for England on the S.S. *Adda*. He did not yet know that Russell, back in New York, had already confirmed that he would return to West Africa in 1930 with a pay raise:

> It is a pleasure to inform you that at the meeting of the Scientific Directors held on December 2, 1929 you were reappointed to the field staff of the International Health Division for the year 1930 at a salary of $4,000 beginning January 1, 1930, and allowance for rent, board, and laundry in lieu of regular commutation while on yellow fever work abroad.[86]

5

Diagnosis Yellow Fever

H ayne arrived in New York on New Year's Day 1930, and reported the next day to Dr. H. T. Chickering at 135 E. 65th Street for a physical examination. He was of "vigorous" appearance, weighed 160 pounds, and had a normal blood pressure. It was noted that he had experienced two attacks of malaria, the most recent in August 1929. An area of his scalp had no sensation due to the nerve injury caused by the automobile accident. Dr. Chickering did not comment on his pulse rate of 100 beats per minute, but did record that the heart "rate changes quickly and when slow a soft systolic murmur is heard at the apex. Not significant if ordinary care is exercised."[1] On January 5, Hayne arrived home at Congaree.

A Short Honeymoon

Theodore Hayne and Roselle Hundley were married on January 27 at St. John's Episcopal Church, Columbia. They returned to Congaree and spent most of the next eight weeks at Wavering Place. Hayne could not afford an extravagant trip. He later wrote that

> I spent most of my vacation riding about the country in the Packard or working on cars in the yard. It did enable me to forget West Africa and the mosquitoes for the entire time and that should be of some help. The time passed like a flash.[2]

A fishing trip with his father never materialized. Roselle experienced a series of head colds.

On March 16, Henry W. Kumm—Hayne's colleague and contemporary in West Africa—sent a postcard from the the Canal Zone:

Dear Ted,

Yesterday at Ancon one of the nurses in the operating room told me you were married. Sincerest congratulations! Do write and tell me how you were able to arrange to take her with you to Nigeria.

Yours as ever,
Henry W. Kumm[3]

Actually, Hayne's situation was the same as Kumm's had been in 1928: The new bride would stay behind.

On March 23, the newlyweds accompanied by Hayne's parents arrived in New York after a leisurely drive that included stops in Washington and Baltimore. Adams Hayne probably provided much of the entertainment, for his son expressed relief that "I was sure glad to hear that you had gotten away from the clutches of the law in the Cosmopolitan City."[4] On March 29, Roselle Hayne and the elder Haynes watched the S.S. *George Washington* slowly leave the New York harbor. In his later life, Adams Hayne found the whistle of a steamship almost unbearable due to the memory of this last glimpse of his son.

Hayne described an uneventful voyage. Drinking was limited to "a weak imitation of lager beer." "The crowd is quiet except for occasional 'I raise you ten.' 'Check it to you.' 'Who can beat these jacks' etc." He thanked his father for loaning the Packard and hoped "that it was not hurt much by my use." He urged his father to repeat the malaria study of the Lake Murray area since it was an excellent chance to study the effect of impounding such a large body of water on the epidemiology of malaria.[5] Hayne had been encouraged to learn in New York that Frederick F. Russell "favors some malaria work being done as well as Y.F," for "Africa needs that most." In the long run, Hayne would be correct.

On April 9, Hayne left England for Lagos on the R.M.S. *Apapa*. He reported a "congenial crowd on board" with preparations for a costume dance on deck. He told his mother how much he regretted leaving Roselle at home; it was "very unfortunate that we could not make this trip together." He expressed serious plans for his career.

He wanted to go back to school, ideally to obtain a doctorate in public health at Johns Hopkins: "Theres a chance of my getting it but depends upon what work there is to be done at that time."[6]

Although Hayne expected that his wife would be able to join him at a later time, the plans were never definite. Hayne told his mother:

> I never did find out definitely what Roselles plans were. I dont think that she knew or had made up her mind. I hope that she soon returns to S.C. and makes herself happy with Susan and Mary. I borrowed most of her money for the trip to N.Y. etc.[7]

He hoped that she might be able to cross the Atlantic that summer with his cousin, Hamlin Beattie. There were three obstacles: lack of money, the reservation about wives at least for younger members of the Rockefeller staff, and a shortage of adequate quarters for married couples at Yaba. Marshall Barber had negotiated for himself a house so that his wife, Nadine, could join him "for a few months, anyway."[8] In January, Beeuwkes had cabled Russell that "Dr. Barber's house will be available by September 1st" and suggested "that Mrs. Hayne defer her arrival until that time."[9]

Meanwhile, there had been a fifth death among the Rockefeller yellow fever researchers. Dr. Paul Lewis, a pathologist who had helped prove that poliomyelitis ("polio") is caused by a virus, had died on June 30, 1929 at Bahia, Brazil. The five deaths had come from a staff that never numbered more than 27 full-time yellow fever researchers.[10] In its annual report for 1929, the Rockefeller Foundation noted:

> Research work in yellow fever, both in Africa and in Brazil, is fraught with great danger to those who undertake it. All honor is due to the scientists engaged in this important but perilous task.[11]

Tree-hole and Crab-hole Mosquitoes

Hayne arrived at Yaba on April 23 and the following day took over the entomology laboratory from Dr. Johannes Bauer. Hayne's assignment was to care for all of the mosquitoes infected with the yellow fever virus. The laboratory was guarded by a triple-door entry system designed to reduce the likelihood that a mosquito carrying the deadly virus might escape. If Hayne was concerned about the danger, he did not transmit his fears to his mother. Rather, his letters beamed enthusiasm. The remaining 79 days of his life would be busy and productive.

He had reason to be excited. Marshall Barber was still at Yaba. Russell had confirmed to Beeuwkes that the "work on malaria in Nigeria seems to me has a great future, and I think we should hang on to Dr. Barber just as long as he is willing to work there."[12] There was the possibility that Hayne might return to malaria research even while in West Africa. Meanwhile, though, he had become interested in the varieties of West African mosquitoes. Barber had caught numerous mosquitoes around the Yaba compound and had given all of them except the *Anopheles* to the laboratory of which Hayne was now in charge. Hayne had the opportunity to become involved in what was then a cutting edge of yellow fever investigation: the role of mosquito vectors other than *Aedes aegypti*.

He began to study "the life habits of certain of the so-called 'other vectors' of yellow fever." Some of these mosquitoes were known as tree-hole breeders and others as crab-hole breeders.[13] These mosquitoes could transmit yellow fever to rhesus monkeys in the laboratory. But did they bite humans? If so, when and where? What were their habits and flight patterns? In sum, were they important?

Hayne found a spot on the Lagos lagoon, about two or three miles east of Yaba, that teemed with the tree-hole and crab-hole breeders. The human population was sparse and scattered. The largest village, Iwonran, contained "about five native houses" with approximately 50 people. There were several smaller villages: Eddu, Odumyao, and Onitiri. What were the interactions between mosquitoes and humans? Could the crab-hole and tree-hole breeders be captured in the houses?

On May 2, after Hayne had been back in Yaba only 10 days, Beeuwkes noted that

> it will be possible for Dr. Hayne to make daily collections to determine to what extent these mosquitoes are found inside

houses. We also plan to make collections of adults, larve and pupae in the tree- and crab-holes. Precipitin tests will be carried out on all blooded specimens included in the catches.[14]

On May 30, Beeuwkes reported that

Dr. Hayne and Mr. Glasounoff have been doing some interesting work in connection with the life habits and flight of numerous species of tree-hole and crab-hole breeders in the village of Iwonran, on the lagoon and approximately three miles east of Yaba. This village of only a few houses is favorably situated for the study as it is in an isolated section with many trees with large and smaller holes breeding *Aedes* mosquitoes of different species. There are also great numbers of crab-holes breeding *A. irritans* and *A. nigricephalus*. In spite of this profuse breeding, Dr. Hayne and his mosquito catchers have not trapped any of these mosquitoes in the houses, and only small numbers of *Aedes aegypti* have been caught.

With a view to securing further information on the flight of these mosquitoes, he recently collected together a great deal of the water from the tree-holes and placing this in a large cage allowed the insects to develop and emerge. By May 28th approximately 150 living mosquitoes were on hand, while a much larger number was found dead on the bottom of the cage. The stock was augmented by many mosquitoes bred at the laboratory and approximately 600 mosquitoes were stained and liberated on that date. These included 200 *A. nigricephalus*, 100 *A. irritans*, 200 *A. stokesi*, 40 *A. apicoargenteus*, 40 *A. luteocephalus*, 10 *A. longipalpis* and 10 *A. africanus*. These mosquitoes were liberated approximately 200 yards from the houses of the village, and though frequent catches have since been made in the houses not a single stained specimen has been collected. At the same time, though the *A. irritans* and *A. nigricephalus* are breeding profusely in the crab-holes, none of these species have been found in the houses.

In order to make a comparison with the flight and habits of

A. aegypti approximately an equal number of this species will be stained and liberated from the cage at the same point within a few days and similar catches will be carried out.

Another collection of the tree-hole breeders will be made, and after staining these will be liberated within sight and a short distance from the homes.

In all catches made to date—including those carried out by former personnel of the Commission and the forces of Dr. Hayne and Dr. Barber—no tree-hole breeder has been found in houses, with the exception of approximately 8 specimens of *A. stokesi* and a relatively small number of *A. nigricephalus* and *A. irritans*.[15]

Hayne briefly described the work to his mother:

During the last two weeks I have been doing a lot of night collecting of mosquitoes on the lagoon about three miles east of here. Its a rather long walk but there are only jungle paths over there unless one goes by boat about five miles from Ebute metta.[16]

It was eventually concluded that "the only proven vector of yellow fever that occurs inside these native houses in appreciable and possibly important numbers is *T. africanus*."[17] But the question remained: if these mosquitoes could not be found in the houses, did they bite humans at all?

Night Catches With Human Bait

Reaching back to his malaria work in Arkansas and elsewhere, Hayne introduced a method that came to be known as "night catches with human bait." John Austin Kerr, a 29-year-old Chicago native who had come to Lagos with Hayne aboard the S.S. *Apapa*, later wrote that

Ted knew that there must be some of the mosquitoes about so he did a very novel thing. Ted may have told you that his personal steward boy had bought a small movie projector. Ted borrowed the movie projector and took it out to the little bush village where he was working and put on a movie show for the natives. They came in numbers. Then, while they were intent on the pictures Ted had his trained mosquito-catchers walk around among the spectators and look, with the aid of electric flashlights, for mosquitoes which were biting the spectators. The boys caught a lot of mosquitoes but the people moved around so much and killed so many of the mosquitoes before the boys could catch them that Ted decided it would be better to have the boys catch the mosquitoes that came to bite the boys themselves.

But, characteristic of Ted, he did not ask the boys to do anything that he was not willing to do himself. When they started on that sort of work, which had to be done at night, for that is the only time that most of the mosquitoes in which Ted was interested bite, Ted went along with the boys. He peeled off his shirt and had one of the boys catch all mosquitoes that came to bite him. They caught a lot, too. But for various reasons that method was not continued, and reliance was placed on what the boys could catch on themselves—which was, after all, quite adequate.[18]

Kerr also noted in his official summary for the Rockefeller Foundation: "On the basis of his [Hayne's] findings night catches with human bait have since been used extensively, and with excellent results."

On June 10, Beeuwkes recorded the "night catches with human bait" in his diary:

A great deal of work has been carried out by Drs. Hayne and Burke and Mr. Glausounoff at Iwonran in connection with the life habits of the tree- and crab-hole breeders. As mentioned, none of the tree-hole breeders have been caught in the houses there, even after the liberation of large numbers of the species, but no catches were made at night. In order to secure further information on their biting habits, Hayne carried over a small movie projector this evening and, while the natives were engaged in looking at the pictures, made catches of the mosquitoes which attacked them in large numbers, and the following insects were caught:

A. luteocephalus	3
Mansonioides africanus	34
A. africanus	6
A. irritans	24
A. occidentalis (or Stokesi)	0

It seems, therefore, that though the tree-hole breeders are very rarely caught in houses they bite very readily, especially toward evening, and it may be actually possible to trap them in the houses when night catches are made.[19]

Hayne showed that of five common tree-hole breeding species of mosquitoes, only two commonly fed on humans. He also established that the preferred time of biting for these two species—*Aedes africanus* and *Aedes luteocephalus*—was "for the first hour or so after dark." Additional studies confirmed these findings.[20]

Although the method of "night catches with human bait" was never published in a scientific journal under Hayne's name, both Kerr and Barber considered this to have been Hayne's major contribution to yellow fever research.[21] Hayne was quickly becoming an authority on mosquitoes capable of transmitting yellow fever. Although his main work was with tree-hole and crab-hole breeders, he had not forgotten *Aedes aegypti*.

The Otta Flight Experiment

Less than three weeks after Hayne's arrival back at Yaba, Beeuwkes recorded that "Dr. Hayne is anxious to carry out some experiments on the flight of the *Aedes aegypti*."[22] Hayne wanted to carry out flight studies using the technique he had learned as a teenager working with Joseph A. Le Prince: spraying mosquitoes with a dye, releasing them, and then testing newly-captured mosquitoes for the presence of the dye. There was a potential obstacle: would the deliberate release of *Aedes aegypti* cause a public uproar?

Hayne carried out a preliminary experiment in Iwonran. On June 7, he released 600 dye-stained, laboratory-bred female *Aedes aegypti*. Over the next three weeks, he attempted to recapture the mosquitoes. Results were disappointing: only 18 female mosquitoes were caught and only nine of these showed the stain. Hayne wanted to repeat the study on a larger scale. Beeuwkes discussed the matter with the Director of Medical and Sanitary Service, who "agreed to let us carry out the work if it were done quietly and at a distance of 15 to 20 miles from Lagos."[23] They chose the town of Otta, located 20 miles north of Lagos and consisting of about 500 houses and 3,000 people.

Later, Beeuwkes recorded that "Drs. Hayne and Burke and Mr. Glasounoff have recently been working in Otta" and "have established friendship with the chief, who assists them in entering homes for making catches and offers no opposition to any work they wish to

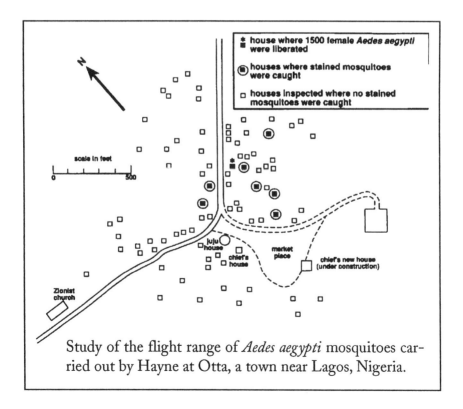

Study of the flight range of *Aedes aegypti* mosquitoes carried out by Hayne at Otta, a town near Lagos, Nigeria.

do."[24] Marshall Barber later wrote that the chief of Otta "was very friendly to anyone who showed an interest in his remarkable collection of native hats."[25]

On June 17, Hayne released 1,500 laboratory-bred female *Aedes aegypti* mosquitoes in an empty house near the center of Otta. Hayne, Burke, Glasounoff, and three native assistants attempted to recapture the mosquitoes on seven occasions over the next 16 days. They caught 1,039 female *Aedes aegypti* mosquitoes, but only 49 of these showed any trace of the dye and of these, 26 were taken in the same room where they were released. Most of the others were retaken in the immediate vicinity. The greatest distance between the place of release and the site of recapture was about 400 feet. Kerr later reviewed the report and found that despite "the large amount of effort expended in this experiment, the small number of stained *Aegypti* retaken make the results inconclusive."[26]

Hayne placed the work in perspective to his brother, Ike:

> I have been recently doing a staining experiment with a lot of Aedes aegypti mosquitoes in a little native village about twenty miles north to learn something of the flight habits of this mosquito in the native village. I released about fifteen hundred well stained and have thus far recovered about thirty of the stained ones. However they dont seem to distribute themselves very far from the point of liberation. This is not a new observation but some recent work done by Shannon in South America caused the Boss here to suggest that we get an idea about their flight habits here under natural conditions in a native village. The houses are rather scattered and it is difficult to keep track of the distance flown because there is no map of the town and the houses are so huddled together that it is difficult to measure back to the point of liberation.[27]

Problems with the experiment may also have included unexpected high mortality among the mosquitoes from natural causes, dispersion over too wide an area, and difficulties with the stain.[28] The results of this labor-intensive investigation were never published.

Hayne's health was ostensibly good and he registered no complaints in his letters home. However, Beeuwkes reported that Hayne had experienced another attack of malaria: "Both Dr. Hayne and Mr. Glasounoff have been spending a considerable amount of time in the bush in making mosquito studies recently and it is possible that they were reinfected there. However, Dr. Hayne had parasites in his blood sometime back."[29] Hayne continued to work without interruption.

"It Certainly Keeps Me Busy"

Hayne took on a third outside project: breeding certain mosquitoes collectively known as "Mansonioides" in captivity. These mosquitoes lived and bred in the root systems of widely-distributed water-floating plants, notably *Pistia* and duckweed. What were their life habits? Could they transmit yellow fever to humans?

On May 22, Beeuwkes recorded that "Dr. Hayne proceeded to Ibadan to collect pistia and duckweed and Mansonioides larvae."[30] Barber had completed his work with *Anopheles* mosquitoes in "the mosquito house which we constructed on the compound for him, and Dr. Hayne will use this enclosure in an attempt to breed Mansonioides in captivity."[31] On May 23, Hayne returned from Ibadan with a large number of *Mansonioides* larvae and a collection of *Pistia* "with numerous larvae attached to the roots." Beeuwkes added:

> He also brought down a cage containing what was estimated to be 800 *Aedes aegypti*. These were checked today and were shown to include 356 female and 268 male *Aedes aegypti*, 15 *Culex nebulosus*, 2 *Culex decens* and 1 *Culex duttoni*. These mosquitoes were caught in two days by six scouts. . . . This work is being carried out with a view to training the scouts for intensive catches of the various mosquitoes in connection with the study of the life habits and in an attempt to demonstrate infection in these insects.[32]

Hayne summarized the project:

> I went to Ibadan on Thursday and came back Friday. Saw Dr
> Walcott and some of my friends from up there and had a very
> good trip. It was necessary to collect a large number of
> Taeniorhynchus (Mansonioides) africanus larvae from the pistia
> leaves that I had found previously there. This mosquito has been
> found in the laboratory to transmit yellow fever as well as the
> Aedes (stegomyia) aegypti but we know little of its life habits
> except that it gets its air from the roots of plants rather than the
> surface of the water. It is not found in the water pots of the
> houses but is found in most of the larger pools and streams of
> the various villages. Dr Walcott also sent down a large number
> of Aedes aegypti that had been caught in the houses of Ibadan.
> The idea now is that we should feed a large number of these
> mosquitoes, that are caught wild in the houses, on normal mon-
> keys to determine whether the mosquitoes have bitten someone
> in Ibadan with yellow fever.[33]

Beeuwkes subsequently commented on Hayne's work with the
experimental mosquito house:

> Dr. Hayne made a very interesting observation in the experi-
> mental mosquito house which we erected in the garden. A large
> amount of pistia, with great numbers of larvae, was placed in
> the concrete basin in the enclosure and, though many adults
> were reared and bit voraciously any individual who went into
> the enclosure, extremely little breeding took place. By careful
> search, Dr. Hayne was able to find a few ova attached to the
> undersurface of the pistia leaves.[34]

This issue was relevant due to "the amount of work that would be
required to eliminate pistia and duckweed from the streams passing
through Ibadan."

Within a short time, Hayne had taken on three research projects:
the life habits of tree-hole and crab-hole breeding mosquitoes; the
flight patterns of *A. aegypti*; and the breeding of *Mansonioides* mosquitoes in captivity. In addition, he carried out protection tests with

yellow fever virus and rhesus monkeys. On June 12, Beeuwkes noted that in order to determine

> whether one or two infective mosquitoes in a large lot secured in Ibadan could be depended on to induce infection by biting, Dr. Hayne exposed two normal monkeys today each to 1 mosquito, and two others to 2 mosquitoes. They were all from a proven infective lot, and Dr. Hayne is certain that all the mosquitoes retained in the cage had originally engorged on an infected monkey.[35]

This work was quite dangerous. Beeuwkes documented that all known efforts were made to protect the workers.

Hayne was receiving regular injections of serum obtained from Dr. A. W. Burke, a field investigator who had arrived in Lagos on May 21. Both Burke and Kerr had experienced yellow fever while working in Bahia, Brazil, the previous year, presumably as a result of working with infected monkeys. Their serum was being studied to determine its ability to protect monkeys from yellow fever. Beeuwkes wrote: "What is more important from the point of view of protection of personnel, we are attempting to secure further information as to the length of time these protective properties persist after small doses of serum, by inoculation of a small number of monkeys with 0.1 cc of serum and determining whether this is still competent to protect after periods of 10 and 20 days."[36] Beeuwkes noted that in a small number of cases, giving serum "failed to influence the course of disease in infected monkeys."[37]

On June 15, Hayne composed a letter to his mother: "At present the mosquitoes and monkeys here are keeping me rather busy but I worry a lot about Roselle. I hope that she is getting along all right and is finding it pleasant at Congaree and Columbia."[38] Plans for Roselle to cross the Atlantic with Hamlin Beattie did not materialize. The cottage at Yaba would not be available for the newlyweds anytime soon, since Nadine Barber enjoyed being in Africa much more than she had anticipated. But Roselle seemed fine with the Hayne family at Wavering Place. As Fannie Hayne wrote her son:

> I have a wonderfully good garden. . . . We have ripe peaches, I
> am going to have peach ice cream and chocolate and caramel
> cake for desert. Roselle had peaches and cream for breakfast.
> Friday Shrimp and Frances had a fishing party for Roselle in
> Charleston on the boat-Lillah, Ike, George & Susan, Crow &
> his wife I'On and Ray and another lady and Dr were in the
> party. They spent all day yesterday on the water but so stormy
> and rough that they could not fish but had a good time. . . .
> They got home last night near eleven o'clock all tired but had a
> good time.[39]

Hayne's sisters had included Roselle in a new bridge club, and their
friends considered her "a grand girl, everybody likes her."

In Africa, Hayne had little time for such diversions as his wife was
enjoying. On June 22, he wrote his brother Ike:

> Besides maintaining all of the strains of yellow fever virus in the
> monkeys and mosquitoes here I have to do a lot of outside work
> trying to study something of the life habits and relative impor-
> tance of the eight or nine mosquitoes other than Aedes aegypti
> that have been shown in the laboratory to transmit the disease.
> It certainly keeps me busy and I seldom get a chance to even see
> what the town of Lagos or the beach looks like. However I went
> to the beach early this morning with Weathersbee and we had a
> swim beyond the breakers.[40]

Albert Allen Weathersbee, 24, was from Ellenton, South Carolina and had come to Yaba as a laboratory assistant on June 4. Nadine
Barber later wrote Hayne's mother that Marshall Barber once in-
vited "just the two South Carolina boys" for "fried chicken and corn
pudding and hot biscuits and cake and ice cream and a lot of other
things a la south" to remind them of home.[41]

Hayne continued to make himself useful in ways other than his
formal assignments. He designed "some new boxes to fit along the
sides" of two Dodge six cylinder cars just purchased by the Rockefeller
Foundation: "I had them made carefully with some good mahogany
timber and then had them varnished with clear varnish and they certainly do look fine."[42]

Hayne summarized his plans and his views on yellow fever to Ike, whom he and Roselle were helping through medical school despite their own limited finances. He wrote:

> The problem of control of Yellow Fever in West Africa seems less and less feasible as we go along. I knew that it was going to take a long time and a lot of money but thought that the fact of our doing some work here might add something to our knowledge of its endemicity and also stimulate the powers of the English government here to do some constructive work in their sanitary program so that in years to come that there might possibly be some control and in the far far distant future possibly eradicate the disease. The flareup of Yellow Fever in South America in 1928 and nine certainly don't encourage us much here. Of course we have attempted nothing here yet in the way of control work and it looks at present doubtful if we ever will. Still they hope to maintain a research laboratory here that will keep going for several years and possibly add something to our present meagre knowledge of this disease. The reason that I think that the English government will not get enthused over its control is that they dont have epidemics too often and their death rate from other diseases is so much higher that it is not the disease of most importance. Apparently the natives have known this disease for so many years that there is some sort of racial immunity and it does not kill them as readily as it does the whites.[43]

He wanted to conclude his work with yellow fever and become active again in malaria control. Barber planned to leave Lagos in December and Hayne yearned that "I certainly would like to work with him again." Yet he indicated to Ike his broad interest in the diseases affecting Nigerians and in tropical medicine:

> There is a lot of Plague in Lagos at the present time and a great deal of money is being spent there to prevent its spread into the interior from the Island of Lagos. Occasionally sporadic cases that manage to slip thru the quarantine occur on the mainland

but they are rather rare. Malaria is of course the most prevalent disease and is quite severe with some. . . . The native children of the various towns and native villages all show a large number of parasites in their blood. One would hardly believe that 100% of all of the children between ages five and ten have been found to have malaria parasites in their blood. The majority have estivo autumnal but many have both Estivoautumnal and quartan. I would say that about fifty percent have quartan in addition.

In Ibadan we found that about seventy percent of the school children of that town had schistosomiasis. Hookworm, Ascaris, tapeworm etc are very common. Guinea worm are very prevalent in certain areas as is also Yaws. Sleeping sickness is on the increase in certain areas and is at present almost wholly confined to northern Nigeria but it has been noted to be spreading somewhat southward in some of the belts or areas. The fly that transmits it the Tsetse is fairly common along the streams here in the south. There is so much disease and the majority of the natives so primitive that it will be a long time before a great deal of work will be done about many of the various diseases. Its a matter of economics. As soon as the produce of the country justifies the expenditure of more money and as soon as the natives themselves are educated to a greater desire to improve their general living conditions and a need for more money these things will come about. The English use all of the revenue of the country for employment of the necessary governmental officers and for the various improvements that are necessary but there is not enough surplus to do all of the medical and sanitary work that they would like to do. I had the idea when I came out here that the Rockefeller foundation would spend a great deal of money in their control campaign as soon as they proved that the disease here called yellow fever was the same as that disease in South America. At present they dont intend to spend any money in control work and feel that their only work here will be to keep the research laboratory going for some time longer. I think that the South American outbreaks of the last three years sobered them down from their world eradication idea. They spent millions in South America and the epidemics in Rio and other places in South America don't seem to show that the control was as good as they expected.[44]

He urged Ike to send him his saxophone; "Shrimp" Hasell was to have sent it, but hadn't. "I cant play it much but it will help to fill in some of the lonely times in the evening. I cant read and study all of the time." His main concern was Roselle. He told Ike that it was "such a shame that there should be any difficulty at all about Roselle's coming out here." He urged his brother to do whatever he could to help Roselle feel at home: "Please do all that you can to keep her from feeling out of place and lonely at Congaree. Im sure that you will tho Im afraid that she feels that she might overstay her welcome there."

Children Are Not Welcome

On June 21, Hayne began a letter to his mother that was completed the following day. His writing may have been interrupted by the arrival of mail that delivered a bombshell. Roselle was pregnant:

In the last mail Roselle wrote something of the happenings at home and the very surprising news that you probably now know of. It was not thought that this would happen before she came out here and I thought even then that it should not prevent her coming but after talking with Dr. Mahaffy it was found that it would be much better that she remain at home until everything was all right. There is so much fear by our director that someone will get sick here and have to be sent home. There is a great deal of malaria. None of the houses of the English are screened and it is a custom that no one dares to allow their wives to stay here after six months. The Doctors at the hospital usually advise them to go to England and practically refuse to do any obstetrical work here in the hospital. There is no milk except canned milk to be obtained for love or money. I would love to have Roselle here but know that her life here would be made miserable by the remarks of everyone about how unwise it was to stay here.

Mrs. Barber planned on arrival to stay only six months but she seems to like it here and wants to stay until Dr. Barber goes to Monrovia in December. If Roselle was all right she could certainly come out in September anyway for Dr. Beeuwkes told me today that everything could be arranged in September for quarters. I have not told him yet for Im waiting to hear from Roselle but feel certain that she would have better care and be in much less danger if she went to a hospital in Columbia.

If I had realized that this would happen so soon Im sure that I would have hesitated in coming back here. Roselle probably thinks that Im the poorest sort of a husband but it seems the only thing to do at present. Please you and Dad both talk to her and try to explain and make her understand.

Naturally Im rather upset and disappointed about her not coming out but feel that we both have more now to think of than ourselves. She will probably find it lonely for a while but as soon as she realizes that we must make the best of it she will get along better.

Im sure that I shall not remain here eighteen months and it is probable that it will not be more than twelve. Dr. Mahaffy says that he is sure that I shall get a malaria assignment somewhere after this tour and possibly after my study leave. This is the only place that we are sent that children are not at all welcome.

Im afraid that Roselle feels that she is imposing on the family to remain so long at Congaree but I feel sure that you and Dad are glad to have her stay there.

It took a lot of sleepless nights to decide whether it was better to stay here now or resign and come home. Please tell Dad to write a long letter to me. I feel that Im doing the right thing but want to be reassured. It must have upset Roselle a lot to receive that cable. I didn't realize that anything had occurred until the last mail arrived. Roselle was anxious to come out in spite of the condition and I was just beginning to learn that such a thing would cause a lot of objections and criticisms here.

Please cable me that everything is all right when you receive this letter.

It seems best that we should go to a hospital in Columbia for that will relieve all of the trouble and worry at home. I think that she would prefer that. . . Next year I'm sure to spend more time at home. It is my plan to stay at Johns Hopkins in Baltimore to take a study course for Doctor of Public Health. The foundation will pay my salary and tuition.

There is a lot for me to do this afternoon. Love to all. Tell the family to write to me.[45]

Hayne had cabled home that Roselle would not be able to come and that he would remain at Yaba. On June 24, his mother wrote him:

Roselle was very gloomy over your cable yesterday and I was just too sorry for her. I could truly sympathize with her, for it carried me back to the first year of my married life when your Dad went in the Spanish war and realized too late that he had a wife and the prospects of a baby, so we were both very miserable over our separation for some months, and especially at that period that I felt I needed him so much. It all seemed so hard and such a useless separation and I grieved very much but as I told Roselle yesterday I felt fully repaid for all my anxiety and trouble by your making us both so happy over your safe arrival to be a pleasure and comfort to us. We were so proud of you and you have fully repaid us for all of our gloomy months we spent before your arrival and I feel sure that where you both feel sad over your separation that it will be only a short time after all and then your lives will be brightened. Altho Roselle is not quite sure she is pregnant—it looks as if so many in the family have been disappointed this summer but when I have so many disappointments I am always hopeful for the best side to turn up after all.

Fannie Hayne added: "Hope you are keeping in the best of health and your stay in Africa will not be as long as you expected."[46] Hayne had casually reported a week earlier that

> Glasounoff who has been working with me got a severe case of malaria last week and had high fever and severe pain over his spleen for about three days. I had mine a couple of weeks ago but am perfectly healthy and normal now.[47]

That would soon change.

"Diagnosis Yellow Fever"

On Saturday, July 5, 1930, Fannie Hayne advised her son that although Roselle was being entertained in Congaree the separation was painful. She expressed concern about her son's health:

> Roselle Lillah and Daisy went to Caughmans pond this morning for a swim. Roselle says she feels so good that she cannot believe there [is] anything wrong with her. I told her she would not feel so good a little later, she is looking well and we all get on nicely and agreeably together, but she gets sad at times over being separated from you and not being able to go over to Africa as she had planned and looked forward to. Of course we are glad to have her and can take the best of care of her. I was in hopes from your cable your tour in Africa will be much shorter and you would soon be with us again. I feel so anxious about your health staying so long in the tropics.[48]

The same day, a group from the Yaba compound went to the beach. Beeuwkes later recalled that "Dr. Hayne was not feeling entirely well. ... He visited the ocean beach at that time but did not go in swimming as was his custom."[49] However, he did not complain. The next morning, at 10:30 A.M., he left with Beeuwkes for Ibadan, where he spent all day Sunday.

On Monday, Hayne and Beeuwkes left Ibadan at noon and returned to Yaba. Beeuwkes would remember that although Hayne did not feel well upon his return, he "worked in the laboratory most of the night in attempting to induce large numbers of *Mansonioides, irritans,* and anophelines to feed upon a monkey which had an especially satisfactory infection."[50] His temperature that evening was 99.2 degrees. Having recently recovered from an attack of malaria, he thought this was a mild recurrence and gave it no further thought.

On Tuesday, July 8, Fannie Hayne sat down to write her son. She felt sorry for Roselle:

> Toli [Frances and "Shrimp" Hasell's young son, Philip Gadsden Hasell, Jr.] is with us. He enjoys staying here for a day or two like you used to at Mamma's . . . I have just made Toli a bed on the floor for him to keep cool and sleep. He asked me who I was writing to, I said to my big boy in Africa. He says "not your boy" he is Roselle's boy. Roselle is getting on fine with all of us–altho at times she gets very blue over the disappointment with not getting to go to Africa as she had planned. I felt so sorry for her and so I did truly sympathize with her, for I never could have a baby that something turned up that I felt was in the way. Roselle looks wonderfully well and says she feels so well is why she could not believe there was anything wrong with her.

She felt anxious for her son:

> I do wish you could give up that work there for I feel so anxious about you for I know you are grieving over Roselle not being with you and I know the separation is terribly hard on you both and I do not feel it is necessary. I think you have already done your bit in Africa and you will find just as necessary work in our own country.

She hoped that her son had received the camera that she and Roselle had purchased for his birthday, and that "you will like it."[51]

The same day that his mother expressed these premonitions, Hayne went to the laboratory but "felt indisposed and tired" after spending the previous night there and returned to his cottage. He spent most of the day in bed. When Beeuwkes and Mahaffy visited him that afternoon, he complained of lassitude, anorexia, drowsiness, "dumbness," and "peculiar sensations between the shoulders and extending slightly down the arms, and he said that his hands felt as if they had been crushed in a vice."[52] He had experienced similar sensations in his shoulders from time to time since his automobile accident. His temperature was 101.5 degrees and his pulse rate 108 per minute. His face, ears, and upper chest seemed congested. The heart was "overactive." Marshall Barber examined his blood for malaria parasites but found none. Examination of a urine specimen revealed "a definite and light cloud of albumin," meaning that there was protein in the urine—a sign of yellow fever although nonspecific.[53]

Although Hayne had received two teaspoons of convalescent serum obtained from Burke on June 25, yellow fever was suspected:

> In view of the nature of the work carried out by Dr. Hayne, the suggestive facies and the mild albuminuria, the case was considered suspicious of being yellow fever. However, as he had had an attack of malaria recently and was taking 10 grains of quinine a day which might have prevented the detection of malaria parasites, even in thick smears, and as his African assistant in the laboratory, who was with him constantly, has just recovered from a severe attack of influenza, several possible diagnoses suggested themselves.[54]

At 5 P.M., blood drawn from Hayne was injected into two rhesus monkeys.

On Wednesday, July 9 Beeuwkes recorded that "Dr. Hayne passed a fairly satisfactory night but his sleep was rather restless and disturbed and he vomited once." His temperature in the morning was 101.6 degrees and pulse 100. The urine was examined twice, at 7 A.M. and 10 A.M., and "both specimens were practically negative for albumin; one showed possibly a slight haze on boiling and addition of acetic acid." Beeuwkes wrote that the symptoms and various findings including Hayne's facial expression "suggest the possibility of yellow fever."[55] Hayne was given another four teaspoons of Burke's convalescent serum, and more blood was drawn from Kerr to be used if needed. At 11 A.M., Hayne was taken to the European Hospital in Lagos. Dr. Gray, the attending physician, "agreed that though the general appearance . . . suggested yellow fever this diagnosis could not be made on the symptomatology or physical signs as the urine remained practically free from albumin and the patient showed no suggestion or jaundice." During the night, Hayne was restless and nervous; the pulse was 90 and temperature 100.8 degrees. Beeuwkes stopped back by the hospital later in the evening and found that "Dr. Hayne is quite comfortable in a large airy room and is receiving every care."[56] On the morning of Thursday, July 10, Beeuwkes went back to the hospital and discussed the case with Dr. Gray:

> Developments during the night inclined him to the diagnosis of yellow fever. The pulse had become somewhat slower without decrease in the temperature. He was restless and nervous and there has been a very slight increase in albumin. In view of this he has officially notified the case.[57]

Dr. Gray seemed to hold

> the impression that Dr. Hayne was much improved this morning and that he will make a satisfactory recovery. The specimen of urine this morning showed only a mild trace of albumin.[58]

Yet Beeuwkes reluctantly concluded:

> The suggestive facies and the slight albumin, together with the marked prostration, indicating a severe toxemia, and the fact that he has been constantly exposed to yellow fever infection would seem to indicate that this is the correct diagnosis.[59]

Beeuwkes telegraphed the New York headquarters:

> HAYNE EUROPEAN HOSPITAL IN CARE OF GRAY DIAGNOSIS YELLOW FEVER MODERATELY SEVERE ONSET COURSE ATYPICAL SERUM 11 DAYS BEFORE BEGINNING ILLNESS CONDITION SERIOUS BUT PROGNOSIS BY GRAY FAVORABLE FEVER MODERATE ALBUMIN SLIGHT NO JAUNDICE MARKED PROSTRATION THIRD DAY HAYNE REQUESTS NOT NOTIFY FAMILY HENRY BEEUWKES[60]

By that evening, Beeuwkes "felt rather pessimistic concerning Dr. Hayne's condition":

He seemed to be nervous and, though entirely rational, he appeared to have an abnormal amount of mental activity to the extent that I thought best to leave him after a short visit.[61]

The temperature remained 102 degrees all day and the pulse varied between 96 and 112. Respirations were somewhat rapid and he was short of breath after slight exertion. He had difficulty swallowing. However, the condition "did not seem to justify alarm." At 9 P.M., he was given sleeping medicine by Dr. Gray. At 11 P.M., the urine showed "albumin equal to one-quarter the height of the column of urine boiled,"an unfavorable sign.[62]

On Friday, July 11, at 2 A.M., the special nurse on duty, a Miss Slaney, "noticed a rather sudden change in the condition of Dr. Hayne" and immediately sent for Dr. Gray. On Dr. Gray's arrival, Hayne "was very restless and thrashing about the bed, but conscious and rational." He was "sitting up in bed and quite dyspenic [short of breath]." His "voice was husky as though he had an acute coryza [viral upper respiratory infection, or head cold]." He coughed considerably and "vomited a small amount of bile-stained material which was not blood-tinged." The amount of protein in the urine had increased, and his temperature rose above 105 degrees. "Emergency measures had a temporary effect" on Hayne's acute dyspnea, but Gray "was not at all satisifed with Hayne's condition." Gray had difficulty telephoning Beeuwkes and therefore "drove out to Yaba and informed us." In the meantime, Miss Slaney was able to reach Beeuwkes by telephone. Beeuwkes and others "were all making preparations to go to the hospital" when they were informed, just as Dr. Gray arrived, that Hayne had died at 4:45 A.M.[63]

An Agonizing Post-Mortem

The Rockefeller Foundation's annual report for 1930 noted that for yellow fever in West Africa:

Only three cases were reported, two from the Gold Coast and one from Nigeria. The one in Nigeria was a laboratory infection.[64]

The Nigerian case was that of Hayne, the researcher who never saw a confirmed case except his own. However, confirming Hayne's case took time. A troubled Henry Beeuwkes would have preferred another diagnosis.

Beeuwkes performed the autopsy himself "for sentimental and other reasons."[65] The latter included reluctance of the regular pathologists and government officials to become involved. There had been no definite jaundice when the autopsy began seven hours after death, but Beeuwkes noted that by the completion of the autopsy "the body, especially the face, front of chest, hands and feet, took on a very mild but definite jaundice tint." Beeuwkes wrote Russell that the gross findings (that is, the observations made on the organs prior to microscopic examination of the tissue sections) were "quite typical" of yellow fever except for the liver which "showed a considerable amount of change" and was "friable."[66]

The heart was "pale and rather flabby." This raised the possibilty that Hayne's lungs had filled with fluid (pulmonary edema) because of heart failure. The stomach showed classic changes of yellow fever, being dilated with "approximately one pint of typical 'coffee grounds' fluid." The lining of the stomach contained numerous hemorrhages and small bleeding spots. Similar bleeding spots (ecchymoses) were present in the duodenum and upper jejunum. The kidneys were enlarged, pale, congested, and "the tubules evidently markedly swollen." There was an incidental but potentially significant surprise finding: a cavity "roughly 2 inches long and 3 inches in diameter" in the apex of the left lung typical of tuberculosis. Most of these changes appeared to be old, but there was some evidence of recent inflammation. This would not have explained the death, but it might have contributed to it.

Could anything other than yellow fever have caused Hayne's fatal illness? There was no history of a mosquito bite in the laboratory or other accident. Hayne was, of course, highly exposed, and could easily have been bitten by a mosquito without knowing it. Also, he had been receiving injections of convalescent serum obtained from Dr. Burke every two weeks, the last on June 25. The possibility that he might have been bitten by a mosquito outside of the laboratory was explored. Immediately after Hayne was taken to the hospital, the foundation's "most expert mosquito catcher, Ali, spent several hours in the house [Hayne's cottage] and did not see a mosquito of any species."[67] The two monkeys injected with Hayne's blood developed low-grade fevers but otherwise remained well, and their blood failed to transmit anything to other monkeys.

The embalmed body was placed in a lead-lined casket which was "sealed again and enclosed in a strong box." Beeuwkes wrote Russell that he was anxious to have "an opinion as early as possible" from pathologists experienced with the disease, such as Paul Hudson at the University of Chicago or Oskar Klotz at the University of Toronto.

Hudson concluded that Hayne had died of heart failure, which was supported clinically by "the short duration of illness (about 4 days), the relatively slow pulse, the clinical signs of cardiac failure, pulmonary edema and the suddenness of death."[68] Heart failure was an unusual way to die from yellow fever, but was not incompatible with the disease. Klotz concluded that the liver, too, had findings consistent with yellow fever. He added: "Viewing the case as a whole we find that we are dealing with a disease inducing degenerative lesions but not inflammation" which was "in itself . . . strong evidence of a yellow fever infection."[69] Klotz found the case especially distressing for he had been at Yaba when Hayne first arrived there: "I took a great fancy to Dr. Hayne . . . and I looked upon him as one of the finest colleagues who had been with us."[70]

The autopsy findings were reviewed by many authorities. S. F. Kitchen concluded:

> We feel that his death was due undoubtedly to cardiac failure and that it was premature in so far as the course of the disease was concerned. We also believe that the large tuberculous focus near the apex of the left lung must have played no small part in influencing the course of the illness. The disease appears to have been quite atypical and gave promise at the onset of not being severe. It somewhat resembled at that time the milder infections we have had here.[71]

Fred L. Soper, in Brazil, received a copy of Kitchen's letter and disagreed:

> Death on the fourth day in yellow fever cannot be considered premature as it is the period at which the greatest number of deaths do occur. The prognosis at any time in yellow fever is most difficult to judge. . . . Personally I feel that a prognosis is difficult to make before the fifth day.[72]

Russell, still director of the International Health Division, reviewed Hayne's file and informed Beeuwkes that the physical examination on January 2 had shown a heart murmur.[73] Russell sent a copy of Hayne's history and autopsy findings to Dr. H. T. Chickering, who had performed the physical examination in January 1930, "because I know that you will be interested."[74]

The Rockefeller Foundation's annual report for 1930 included a note about just how infectious the yellow fever virus was:

> The enormous extent to which yellow fever virus can be diluted and still produce fatal infection in monkeys has been confirmed. A former study showed that a very minute quantity, one millionth (0.000001) cc. was enough to cause infection. More recently it has been found that amounts between one ten-millionth (0.0000001) and one billionth (0.000000001) cc. have frequently proved fatal. The amount of infectious blood, commonly used in the protection tests . . . (0.1 cc), represents approximately one million lethal doses of the virus.[75]

One of Hayne's contemporaries determined that the bite of a mosquito injected at least 100 infective doses of virus to rhesus monkeys.[76] "So far as is known," added Johannes Bauer, "no infective agent has been discovered throughout the course of medical history which, when brought into the laboratory, has caused so high a rate of accidental infection among research workers as has the virus of yellow fever during the past three years."[77]

In the end, all of the authorities concurred that Hayne had died of yellow fever probably resulting from a mosquito bite.[78] The Rockefeller

Foundation now had six martyrs: Cross, Stokes, Noguchi, Young, Lewis, and Theodore Brevard Hayne.

Farewell to Yaba

On Monday, July 14, 1930, a "beautiful memorial service for Dr. Hayne was conducted at the Colonial Church, Lagos, by Mr. Wright, assisted by Mr. Peacock. The small church was crowded." The spectacular flower arrangements included pieces made by Mrs. Beeuwkes and by Nadine Barber. Ruthven Alexanderson Wright, the chaplain, delivered a brief homily:

> My Brothers,
>
> We are here to thank God for the memory of a soldier in the service of mankind who open-eyed faced the risks of his calling and paid the price of our final victory over disease.
>
> Since we are men, we are more than a little distressed that one so gallant should pass over so soon but we must not be sorry as men without hope. If the Faith that Jesus came to preach means anything it means that such a man is very dear to the heart of God, and that he is even now in the presence of Him who also died that he might live. Some men are called to die for their country encouraged by the thrill of battle, this, our brother, no whit less gallantly laid down his life in the quiet of his laboratory fighting a silent and unseen enemy of us all. For the example of his life and the courage of his sacrifice I would have you thank God.
>
> In your prayers this afternoon I would bid you pray for all those who loved him, especially for her who bears the heaviest burden in this sad happening. I would bid you pray too for us all that God may give us courage, like him, bravely to do our duty.[79]

The disposition of Hayne's estate was a simple matter. He was essentially penniless. Beeuwkes noted:

> Dr. Hayne had no funds in his possession as 25 pounds were drawn in April and this had been expended at the time he be-

came ill. He was about to request an advance at the time illness was initiated. Dr. Hayne had no deposit in the bank at Lagos; such funds as he kept on hand were in his personal possession.[80]

Preparations were made for a hermetically sealed casket. The casket "was placed in a large outer case . . . and shavings and sawdust were solidly packed between the casket and the case." Beeuwkes reminded Russell that there were no undertakers in the colonies and that embalming was done after an extensive autopsy. He wrote: "It is imperative, therefore, that the casket should not be opened upon arrival at its destination."[81] On July 18, Hayne's body left Lagos aboard the S.S. *West Kedron* of the American-West African line, bound for New York.

6
Coming Home

I t took 36 days for Hayne's casket to travel from Lagos, Nigeria, to Congaree, South Carolina. Meanwhile, condolences streamed into the Rockefeller research compound at Yaba. The secretary of the London-based Colonial Medical Research Committee conveyed to Henry Beeuwkes

> an expression of deep regret and sympathy in the loss which the Commission has sustained in the death of a worker of so great accomplishment and promise, and from a disease whose mysteries he was at the time of his death engaged in elucidating.[1]

Those who had known Hayne agreed that he "was universally liked owing to his most charming personality."[2] One Lagos official, for example, wrote that Hayne

> was one of the most likeable men I ever met and his loss will be felt keenly both in your social and scientific activities. My wife and I met him first at Ibadan and I shall never forget the bright sparkle of his personality. After that we used to meet him frequently at the Evans. One of my recollections of him will always be his infectious gaiety at a picnic on the beach.[3]

Another reflected that it

> almost seems impossible to associate death with such a sunny nature—the Gods must have indeed loved him to want him so young. One's only consolation in this sorrow is that such heroism and sacrifice is not altogether wasted—it must ever prove a stimulus to the generations that come after for a man to lay

down his life for the good of his fellow men. He has entered into a glorious fellowship with the "Immortals"—can anyone desire more.[4]

On Tuesday, August 19, 1930, Dr. James Adams Hayne and his son Isaac, who bore "a startling resemblance to his brother," reported to the offices of the Rockefeller Foundation. George H. Ramsey escorted them to Pier 38 in Brooklyn. After the *West Kedron* docked at 3:15 P.M., "Dr. Hayne met Captain Nicholson and inspected the ship."[5] On August 21, the two Haynes, Ramsey, and Henry Kumm—Hayne's friend from Yaba—met at the New Yorker Hotel and proceeded to Pier 36, North River. At 10:36 A.M., they boarded the S.S. *Mallory*. Dr. Frederick F. Russell arrived a few minutes later, and Theodore Hayne's body was placed on the ship. The S.S. *Mallory* sailed for Charleston.

Ramsey kept a meticulous diary of subsequent events:

> The S.S. "H. R. Mallory" which sailed at noon is a Clyde Line vessel of 6063 tons regularly traveling between New York and Jacksonville. She is primarily a freighter. There are 78 passengers on the present roster which number is said to be the full passenger capacity of the ship. Dr. J. A. Hayne, who is familiar with the "H. R. Mallory" from previous trips, stated that the initials "H. R." stand for "hell rolling." The behavior of the ship indicates that this may be true.
>
> During the afternoon and evening Dr. Hayne referred to Theodore frequently, and described many events of his boyhood and later life—all of this discussion being without bitterness but showing plainly that Theodore has been almost deified by the members of his own family. Dr. Hayne told us that Theodore's great great grandfather, a Captain Lunsford, died from yellow fever at Columbia during the Revolutionary war.[6]

The next day, Kumm, Ramsey, and the two Haynes played bridge "most of the afternoon and evening." At 6:30 A.M. on August 23, the *H. R. Mallory* docked in Charleston where it was met by Dr. Leon

Banov, the Charleston County health officer, and Theodore's best friends, "Shrimp" Hasell and Hamlin Beattie, along with the undertaker. The coffin was taken to Congaree by motor hearse. Dr. Banov took Kumm and Ramsey on a "sightseeing trip around Charleston, which city is so laid out and semi-tropical enough to be faintly reminiscent of Lagos."[7]

Grief at Congaree

The party left Charleston by Packard sedan and reached Columbia "over 100 miles inland" at 1:30 P.M., in time for lunch. Ramsey described Congaree as

> a railroad station 18 miles from Columbia, but only a station, there being no village nearby. The Hayne homestead is located a mile and a half away from the paved highway, at the end of a narrow road which winds through woods, cotton fields, and corn fields. The house which is about 75 years old is of the Colonial type with six white columns in front, upper and lower verandahs, and very large rooms. It is set in a sandy yard where there are tall magnolia trees, rambling shrubbery and flower beds.[8]

Living in the house along with Dr. and Mrs. Hayne were six daughters and two sons. Three of the daughters were married. There were three grandchildren. Ramsey elaborated:

> All of the family and the husbands of the married daughters were at the house when we arrived. Mrs. Theodore Hayne and her mother who lives in Lynchburg, Va., were also present. Numerous relatives and friends of the family called during the afternoon and evening. These callers included Dr. J. A. Hayne's mother, a spirited and charming lady who is said to be 80 years old, but appears very much younger.[9]

Henry Kumm talked with Roselle Hayne "for a long time and was able to tell her a great deal about Theodore's life in West Africa because the two men were closely associated there." Kumm received a telegram that his own father had died in San Diego, California.

Having seen his father recently and expecting the death, Kumm chose to stay at Congaree for his friend's funeral. At 4 P.M., Hayne's body arrived at Wavering Place and was placed in the front parlor.

On the morning of Sunday, August 24, Kumm and Ramsey toured "the Murray dam and lake, an extensive impounded water project near Columbia," accompanied by "Shrimp" Hasell and the state malariologist. They returned to Congaree for the funeral at St. John's Episcopal Church. Kumm and Ramsey were active pallbearers along with "friends of Theodore Hayne during his boyhood or college days." Members of the South Carolina Medical Association served as honorary pallbearers.[10] Ramsey wrote that the funeral was

> held in a small country church about a half mile away from the Hayne homestead. The body was interred in the churchyard which Mrs. Hayne told me is very old. She also said that nearly all the persons buried there were in some way "kith and kin." The funeral services were conducted by Dr. Williams, the rector of the church, assisted by Dr. Davison Douglas, President of the University of South Carolina. There was no sermon, but Dr. Douglas read the address given at the service held at the Colonial Church in Lagos, Nigeria. The South Carolina church is smaller than the Colonial church, but the color of the walls of the interior is the same. Because of this, the semi tropical setting of the church, and the occasion itself, the funeral of Adrian Stokes came sharply back to memory.
>
> Hymns were sung during the service and at the grave by an excellent quartette from Columbia. At the end of the service the body was taken into the churchyard and final prayers said there. The large crowd of people who could find no room in the church were able to hear the prayers at the grave. The casket was placed in the mahogany box in which it had been shipped from Africa, the grave filled and covered with flowers.
>
> After the funeral, Dr. Kumm and myself again talked about Theodore with Mrs. J. A. Hayne and Mrs. Theodore Hayne. We left for Columbia at 6 p.m.[11]

Appreciation in New York

Hayne's death deeply concerned the small, close-knit group of Rockefeller Foundation yellow fever investigators. From Brazil, Fred L. Soper wrote to Hayne's father that the

> sad news of your son's death in Lagos has just been received in Brazil. I wish you and other members of the immediate family to know that you have the deepest sympathy of the entire yellow fever staff in Brazil.[12]

From Toronto, Klotz wrote to Frederick F. Russell that Hayne

> was a man of great possibilities and a most likeable associate in the work. I took a great fancy to Dr. Hayne when he was with us in 1928 and I looked upon him as one of the finest colleagues who had been with us. He was unusually well adapted for work in tropical medicine and his previous training made him a very valuable man.[13]

In Yaba, Beeuwkes recorded in his report for 1930 that

> the heavy loss which we have sustained in the death of Dr. T. B. Hayne, the loss to science of a brilliant and exceptionally promising worker, and to his colleagues of a true and helpful friend. . . . Dr. Hayne will be remembered by his many friends in Lagos long after the West African Yellow Fever Commission ceases to exist.[14]

For the formal eulogy, the Rockefeller Foundation turned to Dr. Wade Hampton Frost, professor of epidemiology at the Johns Hopkins School of Hygiene and Public Health. Frost, a Virginian who was the son and grandson of prominent Charleston physicians, was the acknowledged dean of the American academic public health community. He had not known Hayne, so he talked to many people, especially Miss Laura Carter and Dr. Louis L. Williams, an eminent malariologist, "both of whom knew him well." Frost confided to Russell:

As nearly as I can ascertain from those who knew him, Dr. Hayne was a man of unusually lovable personality and of very fine character, not remarkable for scientific attainments, but with a somewhat unusual aptitude for field work in malaria and yellow fever. Dr. Carter, as I know from conversation with him and from some of his letters, considered him in character, training and aptitude perhaps the most promising young man that he knew in this particular field, and knowing the esteem in which Carter himself was held by Dr. Hayne's father, I have thought that some allusion to Carter's esteem of young Hayne would be pleasing and at the same time entirely truthful.[15]

Frost presented the resolution on October 14, 1930. After summarizing Hayne's career, he concluded:

From the beginning of his association with the U. S. Public Health Service, Dr. Hayne showed such excellence and stability of character and such aptitude for his work as to win the highest praise of Carter, Barber, and Le Prince and later, of those with whom he was associated in West Africa. A keenly observant naturalist, full of vigorous enthusiasm, steady of purpose, he was recognized by all who knew him as a man of unusual ability; and as a gentleman of high ideals, generous nature, and charming personality, he was universally beloved. His early death is a sad loss to the cause which he had adopted and in which he rendered such effective service.[16]

Such praise did not satisfy Fannie Thorn Hayne. She wanted to learn as much as she could about the circumstances of her son's illness. During those last hours, did he speak of the family? What had he accomplished, and what would become of it?

Nadine Barber's Story

Nadine Barber, who had no children of her own, wrote to Dr. and Mrs. James Adams Hayne from Yaba shortly after their son's death:

Until two weeks ago we were all so happy out here—Like one big family. Nearly every afternoon at 5:30 Theodore and two or three other boys came over to play Badminton or croquet on our lawn and then sat with us afterwards until their dinner gong sounded. He seemed so well and full of life and was making such plans for his wife's coming this Fall.

Dr. Barber and I were delighted when we heard he had decided to return for another tour. Everybody was, in fact, for he was the most popular and beloved man who had ever been here. People often say that he and Dr. Stokes (who died here of yellow fever) were the two best loved members of the Commission and much alike in their enthusiasm and self forgetfulness.

He still seemed like just a boy to me, but Dr. Barber said he had grown so fast mentally and with his tremendous energy (never saving himself enough) he was making a name for himself.

Losing him is a sad blow to Dr. Barber. He had a great devotion for him, as you know—has always had it from their first work together. Since this has happened it seems as if the whole spirit of the place has changed. I wondered for a time if they could carry on, but scientific men are marvelous. They are pulling themselves together and plunging in again. They say this shows how little they know about the disease of yellow fever.

This sounds as if we are thinking only of ourselves in this loss, but I assure you we think of you first in your great grief. Some of the older men said, "Why couldn't it have been one of us who has been so long away from our families instead of a fine young boy like that just married." I believe they would gladly have taken his place and gone out for him if they had been given the chance.

If there is any consolation in such things, it is that he died for a great cause. None of these men out here want credit for bravery or self sacrifice, and he least of all, but it is due them all the more. I think they are braver than soldiers on the firing line.[17]

Fannie Hayne evidently replied and asked many questions, for Nadine Barber wrote again:

> Dear Mrs. Hayne, I wish I could write something helpful instead of all these sad details . . . but you asked for them and it is natural you should want to know. The question pounds through my brain all the time, why did it have to happen and why to him of all people. He is the fourth now of this Commission who has gone out with yellow fever. . . . It all seems to me an awful toll. I myself wonder that they have the courage to keep on, but with each death they seem to realize how little they know about the whole thing and plunge in deeper still. Theodore knew the danger but had so much enthusiasm and the real scientific spirit and the courage to run it down. They all say he was perfectly fearless. What he wanted was results. He told me when I cautioned him about the danger that he was very, very careful. But you see the danger of infection is so great.

She tried to reassure Fannie Hayne that her son had not died among strangers:

> Your dear boy died in a great cause, that is something, and he did not die among strangers or of a long illness, and he died practically in harness doing the work he particularly wanted to do. We all talk about him as if he were still here, never sad any more but just the jolly things. . . . We have the most beautiful memory of him. Nothing can spoil that.

She added a postscript:

> I want to tell you how much the black boys of the laboratory loved him. When he fell ill they all signed a paper and took it to their Mohamedan [Mohammedan] priest, a sort of Ju Ju man, begging his help. He had them get the dirt from one of Theodore's recent foot prints and he wrapped it in the paper on which their names were written and placed it in one of the mosques in Lagos.[18]

Austin Kerr's Story

Austin Kerr, the slightly younger American who had come to Nigeria with Hayne on the S.S. *Apapa*, took over Hayne's research projects. Beeuwkes wrote that

> Dr. Hayne had carried out an enormous amount of work previous to becoming ill, but practically none of his various experiments and studies had been completed at the time of his death. . . . I had frequently impressed upon Dr. Hayne the importance of recording all of his results and promptly reporting them. He had this in mind, but none of his studies had reached a point justifying a report, except several attempts to transmit yellow fever by *A. costalis*. An enormous amount of work along this line was being done by him at the close of his previous tour and further experiments were carried out just before he became ill but, unfortunately, the results are not summarized in any report. Dr. Kerr is taking over this work now but, as he has had only little experience in entomological studies, it will take him a considerable period to orient himself and renew the work begun by Dr. Hayne. We trust that this will work out satisfactorily, but it will require a considerable amount of time before the program can be redeveloped.

On October 9, Fannie Hayne—still pursuing the details of her son's last days at Yaba—wrote directly to Kerr. What had her son accomplished? What would become of his efforts? And did he speak of the family during those last hours? Kerr responded in detail on December 8, apologizing for the delay:

> First of all, I wish to tell you again how very much we all thought of Ted, both on account of his most winsome personality and because of the great energy and ability with which he attacked the various assignments given him out here. It has been my lot to take over the work that he was doing, and so I can tell you of his work at least as well as anybody here at Yaba.

As to the last hours:

> During the first part of his illness Ted was always completely rational and never unduly alarmed. He fully realized that he might have yellow fever. Any of us would realize that. I know I did when I was sick, but I think that caused him no undue alarm or anxiety. At any rate he was what doctors and nurses would call "an excellent patient" all during his illness, and did everything possible to help those that were taking care of him.
>
> In answer to your query as to whether or not Ted spoke of you-all during his illness I am bound to say that he did not—at least, not to the knowledge of any of those who took care of him. But, judging from my own experience—which is, I think, the usual one—I think that can be readily explained. During the first part of his illness, while Ted was completely rational and naturally expected to get well, there was no real cause for speaking of you. But, again judging from my own experience, I am positive that he was thinking of you-all. And then, when the sudden attack that carried him off came on, Ted was much too ill to speak of any one.

Kerr described in detail Hayne's research with mosquitoes other than *Aedes aegypti*:

> The work which Ted was doing is perhaps the most interesting and worth-while of the various problems being worked upon by this Commission. In recent years about eight different species of mosquitoes have been shown to be capable of transmitting yellow fever from monkey to monkey. These eight are aside from the old *Aedes aegypti* which is the classical and most important carrier of the disease. But all the work by which these mosquitoes were proved capable of transmitting yellow fever has been done with monkeys in the laboratory. Now we still have the job of trying to find out just how important these mosquitoes are when they are wild in nature and free to bite the animal they most prefer. Many of these other species are very different from

Aedes aegypti in that they apparently prefer the blood of other animals, and even birds and lizards to that of man.

In the short time that he worked Ted proved that certain of the species which we had shown to be capable of transmitting yellow fever in the laboratory never bit man in nature. One of those mosquitoes is named *Aedes stokesi*, recently renamed in honor of Dr. Adrian Stokes who worked at this laboratory and was the first man to contract yellow fever in the laboratory—in any laboratory. That finding of Ted's is of importance because it eliminates that mosquito from consideration as a carrier of the disease.

He added: "It is a great regret to us all that no one of these things is in such shape that it can be published under Ted's name."[19]

Kerr prepared a 16-page summary of Hayne's observations for the annual report of the West African Yellow Fever Commission. "Most of the work," he commented, "was preliminary and tentative, but it gave some important leads to further work."[20] Kerr later published a detailed article "on the abundance, distribution and feeding habits of some West African mosquitoes." The first table gave data concerning 14,554 mosquitoes caught in 18 small bush villages near Yaba under Hayne's supervision. Kerr credited Hayne in a footnote.[21]

Criteria for co-authorship on scientific papers was much more stringent then than is the case today. Kerr acted properly. Kerr included Hayne as a co-author of an article showing that transfer of the yellow fever virus from female to male *A. aegypti* occurred infrequently if at all.[22] Similarly, Henry Beeuwkes included Hayne on an article showing that trying to capture infected mosquitoes was an inefficient way of determining whether yellow fever was prevalent in a native town.[23]

For 1930, the Rockefeller Foundation's annual report included an obituary of Hayne which read in part:

> Dr. Hayne became a special member of the Foundation's field staff, in June, 1928, and was immediately sent to West Africa to

assist Dr. Beeuwkes in yellow fever studies. His work there was of great importance, both to science in general and to our knowledge of the malady which exacted this grim sacrifice. In his death the Foundation has lost one of its most brilliant and promising workers.[24]

Epilogue
"That's Theodore's Car"

On January 9, 1931, Roselle Hayne, having spent her pregnancy with the family at Congaree, went into labor. She had planned to name the child Theodore or Theodora. The child entered the world with the umbilical cord around her neck—cutting off her breathing and cutting off the family's one opportunity to care for Theodore Hayne's living legacy.

The Hayne family was devastated by the stillbirth and strained by the financial burden of Roselle's extended visit. She remained in Congaree and Columbia for a while but was unable to find satisfactory work. The bank in which she had deposited her savings failed in the Depression. She had problems with her eyesight. The Rockefeller Foundation lent support for which she expressed gratitude for the "generosity in making this allowance for me."[1]

The Conquest of Yellow Fever

Two 1931 developments reduced the risk of yellow fever among researchers: a better animal model and, more importantly, a vaccine. Both of these resulted from an observation that Max Theiler reported in April, 1930—the same month that Hayne returned to Yaba for his second tour. Theiler found that white mice were susceptible to the yellow fever virus when the virus was injected directly into their brains.[2] Previous attempts to transmit yellow fever to mice had failed. Theiler would be the Rockefeller Foundation's Nobel Prize recipient for contributions toward the conquest of yellow fever.

Researchers quickly adopted the mouse model for serologic diagnosis. A mouse protection test replaced the costly, awkward, and probably more dangerous monkey protection test that Hayne had been using up until the time of his death. It was immediately apparent that a "much smaller, less expensive, and more manageable animal will be available as an aid in delimiting the large areas where yellow fever is now occurring in light form."[3] The mouse model enabled rapid attenuation (weakening) of the yellow fever virus so that it could be used as a vaccine. Between May 13 and June 29, 1931, ten persons were vaccinated. The vaccine consisted of an inoculation of attenuated yellow fever virus along with a dose of immune serum.[4] Vaccine was rushed to the small group of highly exposed field workers. At the end of the year, the Rockefeller Foundation noted with pleasure that it "does not have to report any deaths from yellow fever among its personnel."[5]

Despite the effective vaccine, yellow fever would not be eradicated from West Africa. The Rockefeller data suggested "a considerable complexity of factors in the region." In 1932, epidemics of yellow fever occurred in rural areas of Brazil where *Aedes aegypti* could be excluded as a vector. These epidemics were linked to a monkey-mosquito-monkey cycle in the forest, with humans as accidental hosts.[6] "Jungle yellow fever" was now understood. Mosquitoes such as those with which Hayne was working at the time of his death could maintain the virus.

Results of mouse protection tests lent further credence to Hayne's prediction that the "global eradication idea" would not be feasible. In 1934, Rockefeller authorities noted that as

> a general result [of the protection tests] . . . it has now become evident that there are two great endemic areas of yellow fever in the world. . . . One of them occurs in Africa and extends from Senegal in West Africa to the upper reaches of the Nile. The other occurs in South America, and occupies practically the whole of the Amazon Valley. . . . Thus for the first time in history we can envisage with a certain degree of exactness just how large these endemic regions are and exactly where they are. . . . To continue to the end the hitherto brilliantly successful cam-

paign against yellow fever by tracking the disease to its lair in the jungle constitutes an inspiring challenge to workers in tropical medicine.[7]

In April 1934, the Rockefeller Foundation closed the laboratory at Yaba. In November, Henry Beeuwkes received the Mary Kingsley Medal from the Liverpool School of Tropical Medicine for his contributions to the field.

More work with the yellow fever virus in tissue culture and in chick embryo tissues by Theiler, Hugh H. Smith, and Wilbur Sawyer at the Rockefeller Foundation eventually led to a highly attenuated strain known as 17D that is still regarded as perhaps the best virus vaccine yet developed. There was, however, another tragedy. In 1942, thousands of American servicemen received a vaccine combined with a small amount of "normal" human serum. There resulted an estimated 28,000 cases of hepatitis with 64 deaths. Contamination of the serum with the hepatitis virus was ultimately traced to an asymptomatic volunteer blood donor on the staff at the Johns Hopkins Hospital.[8]

Today, jungle yellow fever remains endemic in parts of Africa and South America. In Bolivia, Brazil, Colombia, and Peru, it affects mainly young, unvaccinated men working in the basins of the Amazon, Orinoco, Catatumbo, Atrato, and Magdalena Rivers. It occurs in forested areas in Africa. Outbreaks tend to occur in the savannahs. In 1986, an epidemic of yellow fever in eastern Nigeria caused at least 9,600 cases and 5,600 deaths. In 1987, epidemics in western and northern Nigeria caused some 1,449 cases and 569 deaths.[9] Surveillance for the disease remains incomplete. Research in yellow fever lags behind that in other areas to the extent that it has been called "a medically neglected disease."[10] However, field workers can now confirm the diagnosis within a few hours by using a method known as an immunoglobulin M antibody capture immunoassay.[11] Work toward developing more sophisticated vaccines offers the possibility that eliminating yellow fever as a public health problem is within human possibility.

Postscript

The Rockefeller Foundation and the Hayne family in South Carolina eventually lost contact with Hayne's widow, Roselle. Hayne's relatives continue to ask the haunting question: What happened to her?

For many years, the old Hudson stood neglected in the yard at Wavering Place. When anyone asked, the answer was: "That's Theodore's car."

Several of Hayne's colleagues enjoyed unusually long and productive careers. Marshall Barber remained active as a malariologist until well into his seventies and received honors from many countries. In 1953, he died at 84 in El Cajon, California. Neil Philip became an authority on tick-borne diseases such as Rocky Mountain spotted fever. Henry Kumm and Austin Kerr became yellow fever experts for the Rockefeller Foundation, which they also served in other ways. Philip died at 86 in San Francisco; Kumm at 89 in Newton, Pennsylvania; and Kerr at 90 in Ossining, New York.

Adams Hayne retired as South Carolina's health officer in 1944, at which time he had held the position longer than any state health officer in the United States. In 1953, he died at Wavering Place at age 78, predeceased by five of his nine children. The road on which he lived and South Carolina's new public health laboratory building were named for him. Fannie Hayne lived to age 95, but never recovered from her grief.[12]

Isaac Hayne ("Ike") and James A. Hayne, Jr. ("the Doctor") spent their careers as general practitioners in rural areas of South Carolina. "Shrimp" Hasell spent his career as an engineer and, during World War II, assisted in the control of malaria in Panama and India.

On December 12, 1953, Susie Stevenson Hayne gave birth to a sixth child and third son. Her husband, Isaac, asked if she had picked out a name and she replied that she had not. "If you don't mind," he said, "I'd like to name him after my brother."

Notes

Abbreviations

Several key collections have been utilized throughout the manuscript. These are fully referenced below and abbreviated as noted throughout the text.

WHL

Correspondence between members of the Hayne family was gathered from multiple family sources. This correspondence in original or photocopy is available in Hayne Papers, MSS#813, Waring Historical Library, MUSC, Charleston, SC. *Designated WHL.*

NLM

History of Medicine Division, National Library of Medicine, National Institutes of Health, Bethesda, MD. *Designated NLM.*

RG9, RAC

Rockefeller Foundation Archives, Rockefeller Archive Center, North Tarrytown, NY, Record Group 9. *Designated RG9, RAC.*

NAC

Malaria file number 4266, National Archive Center, Washington, DC. *Designated NAC.*

Prologue: Epitaph in a Country Churchyard

1. Centers for Disease Control, "Update: Human Immunodeficiency Virus Infections in Health-Care Workers Exposed to Blood of Infected Patients," *Morbidity and Mortality Weekly Report* 36 (May 22, 1987): 285-289.

2. Douglas N. Walton, *Courage: A Philosophical Investigation* (Berkeley, California: University of California Press, 1986).

3. William S. Dutton, "Battling Diseases," *Colliers* (May 5, 1951): 66. Dutton does not provide a reference for this statement.

4. Minutes of the Columbia Medical Society for 1930. The South Caroliniana Library, University of South Carolina, Columbia.

1. "Not Like His Father"

1. The elder Hayne signed his professional papers "James A. Hayne" rather than "J. Adams Hayne," but he was widely known as "Adams Hayne" by contemporaries.

2. James O. Breeden, "Disease as a Factor in Southern Distinctiveness," in Todd L. Savitt and James Harvey Young, eds., *Disease and Distinctiveness in the American South* (Knoxville: The University of Tennessee Press, 1988), 11.

3. See, for example, M. Foster Farley, "The Mighty Monarch of the South: Yellow Fever in Charleston and Savannah," *The Georgia Review* 23 (Spring 1973): 56-70; and Elizabeth Young Newsom, "Unto the Least of These: The Howard Association and Yellow Fever," *Southern Medical Journal* 85 (1992): 632-637.

4. Familiar popular accounts include William H. McNeill, *Plagues and Peoples* (Garden City, New York: Anchor Book, 1976); and Hans Zinsser, *Rats, Lice, and History* (Boston: Published for the Atlantic Monthly Press by Little Brown and Company, 1935).

5. William Osler, "The Study of the Fevers of the South," *Journal of the American Medical Association* 26 (1896): 999-1004.

6. Harry Block, "Sir Ronald Ross, FRS, KCMG, KGB, and the Conquest of Malaria," *Southern Medical Journal* 85 (1992): 407-410.

7. H. R. Carter, "Note on Interval Between Infecting and Secondary Cases of Yellow Fever from the Records of the Yellow Fever at Orwood and Taylor, Miss. in 1898," *New Orleans Medical and Surgical Journal* 52 (1900): 617-636.

8. Walter Reed, James Carroll, A. Agramonte, and Jesse W. Lazear, "The Etiology of Yellow Fever: A Preliminary Note," *The Philadelphia Medical Journal* 6 (1900): 790-796.

9. For concise biographies of Lazear, see Emmett B. Carmichael, "Jesse William Lazear," *Alabama Journal of the Medical Sciences* 9 (1972): 102-114; and J. A. del Regato, "Jesse William Lazear: The Successful Experimental Transmission of Yellow Fever by the Mosquito," *Medical Heritage* 2 (1986): 443-452. For an argument that Lazear should receive the bulk of the credit, see Jon Franklin and John Sutherland, M.D., *Guinea Pig Doctors: The Drama of Medical Research through Self-Experimentation* (New York: William Morrow and Company, Inc., 1984), 183-226. The prevailing viewpoint is that Lazear's infection was accidental. Most historians view the work as a team effort to which Walter Reed brought experience, leadership, and insight. It is not my purpose here to take any position in this debate. A recent reviewer concluded that "the credit usually bestowed on Reed must be reapportioned" among two members of the Liverpool Commission (Herbert Edward Durham and Walter Myers) for the decision to pursue the mosquito theory and Lazear for the proof of its validity (Francois Delaporte, *The History of Yellow Fever: An Essay on the Birth of Tropical Medicine* [translated by Arthur Goldhammer, Cambridge, Mass.: The MIT Press, 1991], 89-90).

10. Elihu D. Richter, "Henry R. Carter—An Overlooked Skeptical Epidemiologist," *New England Journal of Medicine* 277 (1967): 734-738. See also Frederick F. Russell, "Permanent Value of Major Walter Reed's Work on Yellow Fever," *American Journal of Public Health* 24 (1934): 1-7; Wilbur G. Downs, "History of Epidemiologic Aspects of Yellow Fever," *The Yale Journal of Biology and Medicine* 55 (1982): 179-185; William B. Bean, "Walter Reed and Yellow Fever," *JAMA* 250 (1983): 659-662; and Theodore E. Woodward, "Epidemiologic Classics of Carter, Maxcy, Trudeau, and Smith," *The Journal of Infectious Diseases* 165 (1992): 235-244.

11. Walter Reed, Jas. Carroll, and Aristides Agramonte, "The Etiology of Yellow Fever: An Additional Note," *Journal of the American Medical Association* 36 (1901): 431-440. The Reed Commission did, however, establish that the causative agent passed through standard bacteriological filters. This is sometimes considered to have been the first demonstration that a virus caused human disease. One erroneous assumption was that mosquitoes that had fed on patients with mild cases of yellow fever would transmit only mild cases of the disease. If verified, "live vaccination" would be pos-

sible. Tragically, three of eight volunteers died during experiments designed to test this hypothesis including the heroic nurse Clara Louise Maass of Bellefield, New Jersey.

12. Standard references include Mrs. Thomas Campbell, *The Hayne Family of South Carolina* (Charlottesville, Virginia: by the author, 1952); and Laura Jervey Hopkins, *Lower Richland Planters: Hopkins, Adams, Weston and Related Families of South Carolina* (Columbia, S.C.: The R. L. Bryan Company, 1976), 370-377. See also Arthur Meredyth Burke, *The Prominent Families of the United States* (London: The Sackville Press, 1908), i, 67-70.

13. For a recent and well-referenced account, see David K. Bowden, *The Execution of Isaac Hayne* (Lexington, S.C.: The Sandlapper Store, Inc., 1977).

14. Robert Lebby, "The First Shot on Fort Sumter," *South Carolina Historical and Genealogical Magazine* 12 (July 1911): 141-145.

15. Fannie Douglass Thorn was born "Frances," but was called "Fannie" by contemporaries, by genealogists, and on her tombstone. The name "Fannie" is retained here, in part, to distinguish her from a daughter, Frances Thorn Hayne.

16. Susan Davis Darby, personal communication.

17. Of South Carolina volunteers for the Spanish-American war, 72.1 percent never left the United States. See Harris Moore Bailey, Jr., "The Splendid Little Forgotten War: The Mobilization of South Carolina for the War with Spain," *South Carolina Historical Magazine* 92 (1991): 189-214.

18. There is no standard biography of James Adams Hayne. On April 16, 1982, the new building for the Bureau of Laboratories of the South Carolina Department of Health and Environmental Control was named the James A. Hayne Building in his memory, and reference is made to the proceedings of that occasion. He was South Carolina's second health officer (the first, Dr. Fred Williams, served from 1908 to 1911). He served in this capacity for 33 years, and at the time of his retirement had been in office longer than any other health officer in the country. Among his accomplishments were the proposal for a state sanatorium (1913); a distribution program for diphtheria antitoxin at no cost to patients; and organized efforts against various infectious diseases and such non-infectious diseases as pellagra. For a critical and somewhat unflattering account of his career as a public health officer, see Edward H. Beardsley, *A History of Neglect: Health Care of Blacks and Mill Workers in the Twentieth-Century South* (Knox-

ville: The University of Tennessee Press, 1987), 142-144. In Hayne's defense, it should be noted that the position was largely a political appointment; that there was no formal training for public health officers in those days (the School of Hygiene at Johns Hopkins, America's first such institution, did not open until 1918); that Hayne seems to have been held in high regard by his peers as indicated by his election to major offices in relevant organizations and by acceptance of his papers in leading peer-reviewed medical journals; and that a letter from Hayne to his eldest son (included in the present volume) suggests an introspective man who was aware of at least some of his shortcomings.

19. James A. Hayne, "The Rights of the Child," *Journal of the American Medical Association* 75 (1920): 143-145.

20. His sisters recalled that "he was very protective of us" (Lillah Adams Hayne and Frances Hayne Hasell, personal communications). He assumed financial responsibility for his brother Isaac's education.

21. This and many other stories are told by Hayne relatives.

22. William Weston, Jr., personal communication.

23. Theodore Brevard Hayne (hereafter, "Hayne") to Fannie Thorn Hayne, December 26, 1906. Hayne sometimes referred to himself erroneously as "Theodore Brevard Hayne, Jr." He was the third South Carolinian to bear this name and grandson of the first, whose son by the same name was born December 24, 1878 and died the next day. WHL

24. The full name was Joseph Albert Augustin Le Prince. Most of his scientific papers were signed "Joseph A. LePrince."

25. Joseph A. Le Prince and A. J. Orenstein, *Mosquito Control in Panama* (New York and London: G. P. Putnam's Sons, 1916).

26. Hayne to James Adams Hayne, June 7, 1907. WHL.

27. Hayne to James Adams Hayne, July 21, 1907. WHL.

28. Hayne to James Adams Hayne, October 26, 1907. WHL.

29. Frances Hayne Hasell, personal communication.

30. James Adams Hayne to Hayne, June 28, 1909. WHL.

31. Ibid.

32. Hayne to grandmother (either Fannie Douglass Thorn or Lillah Adams Hayne), February 6, 1910. WHL.

33. Frances Hayne Hasell, personal communication, February 2, 1991.

34. See Anthony Toomer Porter, *The History of a Work of Faith and Love in Charleston, S.C., which Grew out of the Calamities of the Late Civil War and is a Record of God's Wonderful Providence. Institution Founded by Rev. A. Toomer Porter, D.D.* (New York: D. Appleton & Co., 1882); and Karen

Greene, *Porter-Gaud School: The Next Step* (Easley, S.C.: Southern Historical Press, 1982).

35. For two recent histories of yellow fever as the driving force behind the organization of public health in the South, see Margaret Humphreys, *Yellow Fever and the South* (New Brunswick, N. J.: Rutgers University Press, 1992); and John H. Ellis, *Yellow Fever and Public Health in the New South* (Lexington: University of Kentucky Press, 1992).

36. There is a tradition that Adams Hayne was told that he could have Wavering if he would return to South Carolina (Julian C. Adams, personal communication).

37. Another tradition holds that Adams Hayne had attended a medical meeting in Chicago and that a drinking bout resulted in his being committed to an asylum. Theodore Hayne and Hamlin Beattie, by this account, drove to Chicago to take him home. When they reached the facility, they were directed to the gymnasium. When asked whom they came to see, a custodian pointed to a tall man holding a medicine ball. "Oh him," the custodian laughed, "that fellow says he's the state health officer for South Carolina!" (Julian C. Adams, personal communication). Another tradition holds that Adams Hayne eventually recognized the consequences of his drinking bouts and became, in later life, a teetotaler.

38. Laura Jervey Hopkins, personal communication.

2. Young Malariologist

1. For a brief biography of Carter (1852-1925), see Elihu D. Richter, "Henry R. Carter—An Overlooked Skeptical Epidemiologist," *New England Journal of Medicine* 277 (1967): 734-738. For a brief sketch of Le Prince (1875-1956), whose full name was Joseph Albert Augustin Le Prince, see Patricia M. LaPointe, "Joseph Augustin LePrince: His Battle Against Mosquitoes and Malaria," *West Tennessee Historical Society Papers* 41 (1987): 48-61. For book-length works by these men, see Joseph A. LePrince and A. J. Orenstein, *Mosquito Control in Panama* (New York: G. P. Putnam's Sons, 1916); and Henry Rose Carter, *Yellow Fever: an Epidemiological and Historical Study of its Place of Origin* (Baltimore: The Williams & Wilkins Company, 1931).

2. *Anopheles* mosquitoes were thus named in 1818, but by the late 19th century only about 100 species had been described. By World War II, more than 1500 species had been described of which approximately 200 had been shown to transmit malaria. *Anopheles* mosquitoes vary widely in their pre-

ferred habitats, feeding patterns, and other habits and in their ability to transmit malaria. See Paul F. Russell, Lloyd E. Rozeboom, and Alan Stone, *Keys to the Anopheline Mosquitoes of the World* (Philadelphia: The American Entomological Society and The Academy of Natural Sciences, 1943).

3. H. R. Carter, "The Malaria Problem of the South," *Public Health Reports* 34 (1919): 1927-1935.

4. Geoffrey M. Jeffery, "Contributions of the U. S. Public Health Service in Tropical Medicine: Part II," *Bulletin of the New York Academy of Medicine* 44 (1968): 737-746.

5. For a summary of this period, see Ralph Chester Williams, *The United States Public Health Service, 1798-1950* (Washington, D.C.: Commissioned Officers Association of the United States Public Health Service, 1951), 295-307. The details of Hayne's work during his summers spent with the Public Health Service are largely unclear. At that time, it was not the custom to acknowledge the contributions of technical assistants in published papers.

6. H. R. Carter to L. L. Williams, Jr., April 26, 1925. Henry Rose Carter papers. NLM.

7. Laura A. Carter to F. F. Russell, September 16, 1928. Personnel file, Theodore B. Hayne. RG9, RAC.

8. Some of Hayne's later letters from West Africa indicate a keen interest in the effect of impounding water on malaria which, along with other evidence that he worked with Carter, suggests that he helped Carter in some of these studies.

9. Williams, *The United States Public Health Service, 1798-1950*, 300-301.

10. James A. Hayne, "Importance of and Factors to be Considered in Selecting New Towns for Malaria Control Demonstrations," *Southern Medical Journal* 15 (1922): 368-371.

11. C. H. Bath, "The Practical and Research Value of Mosquito Traps," *American Journal of Tropical Medicine* 18 (1931): 147-150.

12. Williams, *The United States Public Health Service, 1798-1950*, 300.

13. J. A. A. Le Prince, T. H. D. Griffitts, "Flight of Mosquitoes. Studies on the Distance of Flight of Anopheles Quadrimaculatus." *Public Health Reports* 32 (1917): 656-659. The relevant passage reads:

> About 270 *A. quadrimaculatus* and 30 *A. punctipennis* were captured in houses and barns in within one-half mile of the Catawba River on the west side. These were stained with a 1 per cent solution of eosin and liberated from the point selected on the east side. Within 72

hours two of them, *A. quadrimaculatus*, were found in a negro shack on the west side of the river. A third *A. quadrimaculatus* was taken at the same place on the following day. It is worthy of note that a large per cent of the Anopheles originally captured for the experiment came from the cabin where the stained specimens were recovered later. The flight distance was 3,090 feet from the point of liberation, providing the flight was in a direct line, 800 feet of which was over the waters of the Catawba River.

In the memorial to Hayne prepared for the Columbia Medical Society (Minutes of the Columbia Medical Society for 1930, South Caroliniana Library, The University of South Carolina, Columbia, S.C.) it was noted that

> one particularly outstanding piece of work was done in Chester County, S.C., on the Catawba River, in which the flight of the mosquito was determined by staining them with an aniline dye, and afterwards discovering the stained mosquito. It was then proved that a flight could be made of one and one half miles. A stained mosquito was discovered after having crossed the Catawba River, which was contrary to the held opinion that mosquitoes could not cross large streams.

This passage almost certainly represents the work cited by Le Prince.

14. Draft of letter from Henry R. Carter to a Mr. Bruce, undated. Henry Rose Carter Papers. NLM.

15. To what extent Hayne continued to work with Le Prince is unclear. Le Prince became deeply involved in engineering issues related to malaria control. See for example, J. A. LePrince, "Malaria Control in the Environment of the Cantonments," *Southern Medical Journal* 11 (1918): 551–556; J. A. LePrince, "Drainage as an Anti-Malaria Measure," *The American Journal of Public Health* 10 (1920): 120–123; J. A. LePrince, "Engineering in Malaria Control," *Southern Medical Journal* 20 (1927): 480–482; and J. A. LePrince, "Historical Review of Development of Control of Disease-Bearing Mosquitoes," *Transactions of the American Society of Civil Engineers* 92 (1928): 1313–1314.

16. Memorial to Dr. Theodore Brevard Hayne. Minutes of the Columbia Medical Society for 1930. The South Caroliniana Library.

17. Fragment of an undated letter to an unknown addressee in the possession of Dr. Julian C. Adams.

18. Landon C. Bell to Hayne, September 21, 1916. WHL.

19. The Citadel Class of 1923, *After Fifty Years: The Citadel Class of 1923 Looks Back* (The Citadel Class of 1923: privately published, 1973). Lack of stringency of admission requirements resulted in a high drop-out rate. Of 133 cadets admitted in 1919, only 47 obtained diplomas on schedule four years later.

20. O.J. Bond, *The Story of The Citadel* (Richmond: Garrett and Massie, 1936), 36. For additional information on the impact of yellow fever on The Citadel during the 1850s and 1860s, see Foster M. Farley, "The Mighty Monarch of the South: Yellow Fever in Charleston and Savannah," *The Georgia Review* 27 (Spring 1973): 56–70.

21. J. B. Hart, editor-in-chief, *The Citadel: The Military College of South Carolina, History of the Class of 1919* (Charleston, S.C.: The Citadel Print Shop, 1969), 174.

22. *Flying Officers of the USN* (Washington, D.C.: Naval Aviation War Book Committee, 1919).

23. Hayne to Frances Thorn Hayne, October 11, 1918. WHL.

24. Hayne to grandmother (either Fannie Douglass Thorn or Lillah Adams Hayne), October 19, 1918. WHL.

25. Hayne to grandmother (Fannie Douglass Thorn or Lillah Adams Hayne), November 8, 1918. WHL.

26. O. J. Bond (to Theodore B. Hayne), undated. WHL.

27. Philip Gadsden Hasell to Frances Thorn Hayne, January 12, 1920. WHL.

28. Philip Gadsden Hasell to Frances Thorn Hayne, undated [probably January 1920]. WHL.

29. James Adams Hayne had just completed terms as president of the Southern Medical Association (1918) and the South Carolina Medical Association (1919). In his presidential address to the latter organization, he had spoken eloquently on "Plagues and Pestilences." He was president-elect of the Columbia Medical Society and of the South Carolina Public Health Association. He was launching his diphtheria treatment project to make South Carolina "the first state in the Union . . . to distribute antitoxin free to rich and poor, black and white alike." See James A. Hayne, "Reduction of Mortality Through Free Distribution of Diphtheria Antitoxin," *Southern Medical Journal* 14 (1921): 785–787; and James A. Hayne, "Problems in the Control of Diphtheria," *Journal of the American Medical Association* 81 (1923): 2073–2076.

30. H. R. Carter to Hayne, February 27, 1920. It seems plausible that Hayne had written Carter about his academic difficulties. WHL.

31. *The Sphinx—1920* (Charleston, S. C.: The Corps of Cadets, The Citadel, 1920).

32. Ibid.

33. Ibid.

34. Fricks to Cummings (telegram), June 29, 1920. NAC.

35. M. A. Barber, "The History of Malaria in the United States," *Public Health Reports* 44 (1929): 2575-2587.

36. Using this device, Barber showed that a single anthrax bacillus could cause the disease in a mouse. When the great German bacteriologist Robert Koch visited the United States in 1907, he is said to have asked to see two specific things. One of these was the organisms (now known as rickettsia) that had been found to cause Rocky Mountain spotted fever. The other was Marshall Barber's micro-manipulator. See Ralph H. Major, *An Account of the University of Kansas School of Medicine* (Kansas City: University of Kansas Endowment Association, 1968), 5. For documentation of Barber's background in public health, see also Thomas Neville Bonner, *The Kansas Doctor: A Century of Pioneering* (Lawrence: University of Kansas Press, 1959), 139. That Barber was also an accomplished storyteller is apparent from such contributions to the *University of Kansas Graduate Magazine* as "On the Recollections of a Hired Hand" (March 1905): 200-211; "On the Biography of Peter the Wise and the Dictionary" (February 1906): 165-167; "The Boarding Clubs of the University" (March 1906): 210-217; and "An Igorrote Dog Market at Baguio" (June 1912): 329-331.

37. Marshall A. Barber, *A Malariologist in Many Lands* (Lawrence, Kansas: University of Kansas Press, 1946), 34.

38. Marshall A. Barber, biographical file. Collection RF, RG9, RAC.

39. W. A. Sawyer to F. L. Soper, August 9, 1939. Personnel file, Marshall A. Barber (3). RG9, RAC.

40. Barber, *A Malariologist in Many Lands*, 15. Barber and Hayne found to their surprise that the parasite index was lower among school children within the rice-growing area compared to those outside of it.

41. M. A. Barber and T. B. Hayne, "Some Notes on the Relation of Domestic Animals to Anopheles," *Public Health Reports* 39 (1924): 139-144.

42. The author of this suggestion received a polite reply from the Assistant Surgeon General to the effect that this idea had been previously considered (R. R. Ruella to Bureau of Public Health, June 13, 1923, and A. M. Stimson to R. R. Ruella, June 19, 1923). NAC. Actually, use of oil was by then unnecessary because of Barber and Hayne's discovery.

43. Greer Williams, *The Plague Killers* (New York: Charles Scribner's Sons, 1969), 120. Williams does not reference this statement.

44. M. A. Barber and T. B. Hayne, "Arsenic as a Larvicide for Anopheline Larvae," *Public Health Reports* 26 (1921): 3027-3034. Paris green is a copper aceto arsenite—a double salt of copper metaarsenite and copper acetate. Within the guts of larvae, it was highly toxic. However, because it had no effect on mosquito eggs or pupae, it had to be applied more frequently than oil.

45. Ibid.

46. Geoffrey M. Jeffrey, "Contributions of the U. S. Public Health Service in Tropical Medicine: Part II," *Bulletin of the New York Academy of Medicine 44* (1968): 737-746.

47. L. D. Fricks to J. W. Schereschewsky, July 1, 1921. NAC.

48. Hayne's precarious financial situation is suggested by correspondence pertaining to the expenses for returning home to Congaree, S.C., from Camilla, Georgia in 1921. Hayne had assumed that the trip would be at government expense, since he had always been reimbursed for returning home from his previous temporary assignments. However, he was advised that this policy did not apply to travel following resignation from a permanent position. Hayne's appeals through the proper channels were to no avail. His superior pleaded with the surgeon general's office that "if not inconsistent, authority be granted making allowance for reimbursement of travel expenses incurred by Mr. Hayne in traveling from Camilla, Georgia, to Congaree, South Carolina." The Assistant Surgeon General denied Hayne the reimbursement because "of the attitude of the Department in the matter of retroactive orders." It seems possible that Hayne's having to bear this expense contributed to his being unable to attend medical school at that time. (See Fricks to The Surgeon General, September 15, 1921, and Schereschewsky to Fricks, September 29, 1921, NAC.)

49. Fricks to The Surgeon General, U.S. Public Health Service, March 27, 1922. NAC.

50. M. A. Barber and T. B. Hayne, "Some Observations on the Dispersal of Adult Anopheles," *Public Health Reports* 39 (1924): 195-203. To study the behavior of *Anopheles* mosquitoes in the Arkansas rice country, they studied flight patterns using the methods developed by Le Prince. They captured mosquitoes at their resting places, stained them, and then attempted to recapture them at distant sites. Near Stuttgart, for example, mosquitoes rested in barns and "in privies, hollow stumps and trees, under bridges, and in the other usual resting places." However, most of the mos-

quitoes at such resting places were gone within six days even though *Anopheles* mosquitoes could live up to 25 days in midsummer.

51. M. A. Barber, W. H. W. Komp, and T. B. Hayne, "Some Observations on the Winter Activities of Anopheles in Southern United States," *Public Health Reports* 39 (1924): 231-246. The winter activities of *Anopheles* mosquitoes were studied in Mitchell County, Georgia; in Escambia County, Alabama; and in Arcadia Parish, Louisiana. It was determined that ova, larvae, and pupae developed in winter just as they did in summer, but at slower rates. Winter-breeding *Anopheles* might supplement overwintering adults in repopulating the area.

52. M. A. Barber, W. H. W. Komp, and T. B. Hayne, "The Significance of the Proportion of Sexes Found among Anopheles in Various Resting Places," *Public Health Reports* 40 (1925): 105-110. It was thought that "the presence of a large proportion of males among *Anopheles* in a daytime resting place indicates nearness to a breeding place." Barber, Komp, and Hayne found that "the more accessible the source of blood, the larger the percentage of females." Distance from a breeding site had nothing to do with the sex distribution.

53. See W. Curtis Worthington, Jr., "A Study in Post-Flexner Survival. The Medical College of the State of South Carolina, 1913," *JAMA* 226 (1991): 981-984.

54. Hayne to Isaac Hayne, March 28, 1929. WHL.

55. Hayne to Katherine Faust, February 2, 1927. WHL.

56. Fannie Thorn Hayne to Isaac Hayne, February 1, 1924. WHL.

57. Hayne to Isaac Hayne, March 25, 1924. WHL.

58. M. A. Barber and T. B. Hayne, "Water Hyacinth and the Breeding of Anopheles," *Public Health Reports* 40 (1925): 2557-2562. Water hyacinth was widely used as an ornamental plant for aquaria and artificial ponds. However, its tendency to transgress desired boundaries made it an agricultural pest. Also, it obstructed navigation, interfered with fisheries, endangered bridges, and polluted water. Barber and Hayne confirmed their prediction that water hyacinth provided a haven for mosquitoes.

59. M. A. Barber, W. H. W. Komp, and T. B. Hayne, "The Susceptibility of Malaria Parasites and the Relation to the Transmission of Malaria of the Species of Anopheles Common in the Southern United States," *Public Health Reports* 42 (1927): 2487-2502.

60. M. A. Barber, W. H. W. Komp, and T. B. Hayne, "Malaria in the Prairie Rice Regions of Louisiana and Arkansas," *Public Health Reports* 41 (1926): 2527-2549.

61. M. A. Barber, W. H. W. Komp, and T. B. Hayne, "Prevalence of Malaria (1925) in Parts of Delta of Mississippi and Arkansas: Economic Conditions," *Southern Medical Journal* 19 (1926): 373–377. Barber, Komp, and Hayne examined blood films obtained from 522 nonselected persons on several plantations, and determined the prevalence of malaria to be four to six percent. Rates had been 17 percent for whites and 22 percent for blacks in similar areas nine years earlier. They suggested that one factor for the decline was an improving economy. They noted, for instance, that 12 percent of the people owned automobiles.

62. Barber, *A Malariologist in Many Lands*, 23. Changing agricultural practices during this period included better draining methods; clearing woodlands; cultivating rice on almost treeless prairies; and flooding the rice fields.

63. T. B. Hayne, "A House-to-House Survey of Malaria in the Missisippi Delta," *Southern Medical Journal* 20 (1927): 474–475. Hayne visited 95 white families (579 persons) and 205 black families (1,280 persons) but found only one case of active malaria. He made malaria smears on 202 apparently well people and found that 15 persons (seven percent) were parasite carriers. He concluded that the prevalence of malaria had declined, even if he might have missed some cases. At least some screening was present in 56 percent of the houses. Automobiles were present in 117 of 277 yards.

64. Ironically, three of the six questions on Hayne's senior examination in medicine would be relevant to his own fatal illness and the discussions that followed five years later: the criteria for diagnosis of pulmonary tuberculosis; the differential diagnosis of continued fever and making the diagnosis of malaria; and the significance of a systolic murmur at the apex.

65. Hayne to Katherine Faust, February 2, 1927. WHL.

66. Hayne to Katherine Faust, July 11, 1927. WHL.

67. The Health Department of the Panama Canal, at Ancon, Canal Zone: *Ancon Hospital* (Mt. Hope, Canal Zone: The Panama Canal Press, 1923), 1–5. Although the hospital was still commonly known as "Ancon Hospital," it was "Gorgas Hospital" on Hayne's certficiate.

68. Hayne to Katherine Faust, July 11, 1927. WHL.

69. Hayne to Fannie Thorn Hayne, November 24, 1927. WHL.

70. Hayne to James Adams Hayne, December 18, 1927. WHL.

71. Hayne to Fannie Thorn Hayne, March 3, 1928. WHL.

72. Hayne to Fannie Thorn Hayne, November 24, 1927. WHL.

73. Hayne to Katherine Faust, October 12, 1927. WHL.

74. Hayne to James Adams Hayne, December 18, 1927. WHL.

75. Hayne to Fannie Thorn Hayne, November 28, 1927. WHL.
76. Julia Courtenay Campbell, personal communication.
77. Hayne to Fannie Thorn Hayne, November 24, 1927. WHL.
78. Hayne to James Adams Hayne, December 18, 1927. WHL.
79. Hayne to John A. Ferrell, January 15, 1928. Personnel file, Theodore B. Hayne, RAC.
80. Ferrell to Hayne, January 29, 1928. Personnel file, Theodore B. Hayne, RAC.
81. Hayne to Ferrell, February 14, 1928. Personnel file, Theodore B. Hayne, RAC.
82. Ferrell to Hayne, February 24, 1928. Personnel file, Theodore B. Hayne, RAC.
83. Ferrell to Hayne, March 24, 1928. Personnel file, Theodore B. Hayne, RAC.
84. Hayne to Fannie Thorn Hayne, March 3, 1928. WHL.
85. Lewis B. Bates to Russell, February 9, 1928. Personnel file, Theodore B. Hayne, RAC.
86. Russell to Henry Beeuwkes, June 5, 1928. Personnel file, Theodore B. Hayne, RAC.

3. To Beard the Lion

1. For fuller accounts of this era, see George K. Strode, "Costs and Manpower," in George K. Strode, ed., *Yellow Fever* (New York: McGraw-Hill Book Company, Inc., 1951), 631-639; and Raymond B. Fosdick, *The Story of the Rockefeller Foundation* (New York: Harper & Brothers, Publishers, 1952), 58-70. See also Wilbur G. Downs, "The Story of Yellow Fever Since Walter Reed," *Bulletin of the New York Academy of Medicine* 44 (1968): 721-727; and John Z. Bowers and Edith E. King, "The Conquest of Yellow Fever: The Rockefeller Foundation," *The Journal of the Medical Society of New Jersey* 78 (1981): 539-541.

2. John B. Blake, "Yellow Fever in Eighteenth Century America," *Bulletin of the New York Academy of Medicine* 44 (1968): 673-686.

3. There are numerous accounts of the devastation wrought by yellow fever in the Caribbean. The first well-described epidemic seems to have occurred in the Yucatan in 1648. Admiral Vernon's 1741 attempt to conquer Mexico and Peru reputedly failed because all but 7,000 of the 27,000 troops were lost to yellow fever. Similarly, General Charles Leclerc's 1802 attempt to conquer Haiti and the Mississippi reputedly failed because of

29,000 deaths out of 33,000 men (J. D. Gillett, *Mosquitoes* [London: Weidenfeld and Nicolson, 1971], 197). Although diagnosis was imprecise and statistics may be arguable, the impact of the disease during this period is beyond dispute.

4. John Duffy, "Yellow Fever in the Continental United States During the Nineteenth Century," *Bulletin of the New York Academy of Medicine* 44 (1968): 687-701.

5. J. C. Nott, "Yellow Fever Contrasted with Bilious Fever: Reasons for Believing it is a Disease Sui Generis—Its Mode of Propagation—Remote Cause—Probable Insect or Animalcular origin, &c." *New Orleans Medical and Surgical Journal* 4 (1848): 563-601.

6. Wilbur G. Downs, "Yellow Fever and Josiah Clark Nott," *Bulletin of the New York Academy of Medicine* 50 (1974): 499-508. For a recent biography of Nott, see Reginald Horsman, *Josiah Nott of Mobile: Southerner, Physician, and Racial Theorist* (Baton Rouge: Louisiana State University Press, 1987).

7. At the time of Reed's discovery, the mosquito now known as *Aedes aegypti* was called *Stegomyia fasciata*. The last epidemic of yellow fever in the United States occurred in New Orleans in 1905.

8. The yellow fever virus is currently classified as a flavivirus. Viruses, by definition, contain either RNA (ribonucleic acid) or DNA (deoxyribonucleic acid) but not both. The yellow fever virus is an RNA virus.

9. Fosdick, *The Story of the Rockefeller Foundation*, 1-29.

10. The appellations were: International Health Commission (1913-1916); International Health Board (1916-1927); and International Health Division (1927 onward). For nearly four decades, the Rockefeller Foundation spearheaded efforts to control diseases and improve health around the world—a role later assumed by the publicly-funded World Health Organization.

11. Fosdick, *The Story of the Rockefeller Foundation*, 59.

12. Strode, *Yellow Fever*, 13-14.

13. The standard biography is Gustav Eckstein, *Noguchi* (New York: Harper & Brothers, 1931). For recent discussion, see Sachi Sri Kantha, "Hideyo Noguchi's Research on Yellow Fever (1918-1928) in the Pre-Electron Microscopic Era," *Kitasato Archives of Experimental Medicine* 62 (1989): 1-9.

14. Yellow fever resembles other epidemic diseases (influenza or "flu" is a good example) in that it is relatively easy to identify an epidemic once it has occurred yet difficult to diagnose individual cases with certainty on

clinical grounds alone. When the first cases of yellow fever appeared in seaport cities, clinicians often disagreed violently and even staked their reputations on the diagnosis: Was it yellow fever or something else?

The Reed Commission had shown that the agent—although unidentified—could pass through a bacteriologic filter that should have easily excluded a spirochete. It seems remarkable that Noguchi would have been so confident on the basis of a handful of cases and even more remarkable that Carter, Gorgas, and other experts accepted Noguchi's explanation without more rigorous examination.

15. H. R. Carter, "The Mechanism of the Spontaneous Elimination of Yellow Fever from Endemic Centres," *Annals of Tropical Medicine and Parasitology* 13 (1919): 299-311.

16. W. C. Gorgas, H. R. Carter, and T. C. Lyster, "Yellow Fever: its Distribution and Control in 1920," *Southern Medical Journal* 13 (1920): 873-880.

17. T. F. Hewer, "The Discovery of Yellow Fever in Central Africa," *Journal of the Royal College of Physicians of London* 21 (1987): 199-201.

18. Yellow Fever—West Africa. Annual Report—1925. RG5, IHB/D. Series 3. Reports, routine. Box 214. RAC.

19. The Rockefeller Foundation, *Annual Report, 1926* (New York: The Rockefeller Foundation, 1926), 224.

20. The Rockefeller Foundation, *Annual Report, 1929* (New York: The Rockefeller Foundation, 1929), 50.

21. Personnel file, Henry Beeuwkes. RG9, RAC.

22. The Rockefeller Foundation, *Annual Report, 1926*, 226.

23. The Rockefeller Foundation, *Annual Report, 1926*, 41.

24. Yellow Fever, West Africa. Annual Report, 1926. RG5, IHB/9. Series 3. Reports, routine. Box 214. RAC.

25. W. A. Sawyer, "The History of Yellow Fever Since the New Orleans Epidemic of 1905," *Southern Medical Journal* 25 (1932): 291-296.

26. Ibid.

27. Adrian Stokes, Johannes H. Bauer, and N. Paul Hudson, "Experimental Transmission of Yellow Fever to Laboratory Animals," *American Journal of Tropical Medicine* 8 (1928): 103-164.

28. The Rockefeller Foundation, *Annual Report, 1927* (New York: The Rockefeller Foundation, 1927), 27.

29. Johannes H. Bauer and N. Paul Hudson, "The Incubation Period of Yellow Fever in the Mosquito," *Journal of Experimental Medicine* 48 (1928): 147-153.

30. Johannes H. Bauer and N. Paul Hudson, "Passage of the Virus of Yellow Fever through the Skin," *American Journal of Tropical Medicine* 8 (1928): 371-378.

31. N. Paul Hudson, "The Pathology of Experimental Yellow Fever in the *Macacus rhesus*. I. Gross Pathology," *The American Journal of Pathology* 4 (1928): 395-429.

32. Johannes H. Bauer, "Transmission of Yellow Fever by Mosquitoes Other than *Aedes aegypti*," *American Journal of Tropical Medicine* 8 (1928): 261-282.

33. Fourth Annual Report, West African Yellow Fever Commission, 1928. RG5, IHB/D. Series 3. Reports, routine. Box 215. RAC.

4. "A Most Satisfactory Man"

1. Laura A. Carter to Russell. Personnel file, Theodore B. Hayne, RAC. In June 1929, Hayne wrote his mother that he had "completed the payment of $2200" and that the following month's salary would pay the interest (Hayne to Fannie Thorn Hayne, June 27, 1929. WHL). Hence, it would seem that he spent $183.33, or 63% of his salary toward repaying the loan.

2. Fourth Annual Report, West African Yellow Fever Commission, 1928. RG5, IHB/D. Series 3. Reports, routine. Box 215. RAC.

3. Hayne to Lillah Adams Hayne, October 7, 1928. WHL.

4. Hayne to Philip Gadsden Hasell, November 2, 1928. WHL.

5. Hayne to Lillah Adams Hayne, October 7, 1928. WHL.

6. Ibid.

7. Hayne to Philip Gadsden Hasell, November 2, 1928. WHL.

8. Ibid.

9. Beeuwkes to Russell, August 29, 1928. Personnel file, Theodore B. Hayne, RAC.

10. Hayne to Lillah Adams Hayne, October 7, 1928.

11. Beeuwkes to Russell, November 1, 1928. Personnel file, Theodore B. Hayne, RAC.

12. Barber, *A Malariologist in Many Lands*, 72.

13. The Rockefeller Foundation, *Annual Report, 1930* (New York: The Rockefeller Foundation, 1930), 33. It was also correctly theorized that mild cases of yellow fever might occur among the children.

14. Yellow Fever—West Africa. Annual Report—1925. RG5, IHB/D. Series 3. Reports, routine. Box 214. RAC.

15. The Rockefeller Foundation, *Annual Report, 1926* (New York: The Rockefeller Foundation, 1926), 42-43.

16. The Rockefeller Foundation, *Annual Report, 1927* (New York: The Rockefeller Foundation, 1927), 31-32.

17. Yellow Fever—West Africa. Annual Report—1925. RAC.

18. Hayne to Lillah Adams Hayne, October 7, 1928. WHL.

19. Hayne to Isaac Hayne, November 8, 1928. WHL.

20. Hayne to Philip Gadsden Hasell, November 2, 1928. WHL.

21. Hayne to Isaac Hayne, November 8, 1928. WHL.

22. Thomas H. G. Aitken, "Henry William Kumm, 1901-1991," *Journal of the American Mosquito Control Association* 7 (1991): 673-674.

23. West African Yellow Fever Commission. Diary—Henry Beeuwkes—1929, January 3, 1929. RG 1.1, Series 495. Sub-series West African Region. Box 5. Folder 31. RAC. Hereafter referred to as "Diary—Henry Beeuwkes," RAC.

24. Diary—Henry Beeuwkes, January 14, 1929, RAC.

25. Diary—Henry Beeuwkes, January 23, 1929, RAC.

26. Hayne to Fannie Thorn Hayne, March 17, 1929. WHL.

27. Hayne to Fannie Thorn Hayne, July 12, 1929. WHL.

28. Hayne's colleague Henry W. Kumm later reviewed this subject. See Henry W. Kumm, "Periodicity in the Annual Incidence of Reported Cases of Yellow Fever During the Past Fifty Years," *American Journal of Tropical Medicine and Hygiene* 1 (1952): 210-219.

29. Fifth Annual Report, West African Yellow Fever Commission, 1929, p. 28. RAC. Official reports of the League of Nations for 1929 indicated 22 cases of yellow fever in all of Africa; all of these cases occurred in Liberia. In Ibadan, Hayne participated in an experiment that shed some light on this observation. Ten rhesus monkeys were placed in cages and observed. None developed yellow fever, suggesting that large numbers of virus-infected mosquitoes were not circulating at least in that area of Ibadan. On October 29, 1929, the monkeys were challenged with the yellow fever virus strain used for the protection tests. All of the monkeys died, confirming that they had been susceptible to the disease.

30. The Rockefeller Foundation, *Annual Report, 1929* (New York: The Rockefeller Foundation, 1929), 46, 49.

31. Hayne to Fannie Thorn Hayne, May 9, 1929. WHL.

32. Hayne to Fannie Thorn Hayne, November 26, 1928. WHL.

33. Hayne to Fannie Thorn Hayne, January 19, 1929. WHL.

34. Diary—Henry Beeuwkes, January 23, 1929. RAC.

35. Hayne to Fannie Thorn Hayne, March 17, 1929. WHL

36. Diary—Henry Beeuwkes, May 13, 1929, RAC.

37. Diary—Henry Beeuwkes, May 14, 1929, RAC.

38. Diary—Henry Beeuwkes, May 26, 1929, RAC.

39. Hayne to Fannie Thorn Hayne, June 2, 1929. WHL.

40. Hayne to Fannie Thorn Hayne, June 19, 1929. WHL.

41. Hayne to Fannie Thorn Hayne, June 30, 1929. WHL.

42. Ibid.

43. Russell to Beeuwkes, July 11, 1929. Personnel file, Theodore B. Hayne, RAC.

44. Russell to Hayne, July 22, 1929. Personnel file, Theodore B. Hayne, RAC.

45. Beeuwkes to Russell, July 4, 1929. Personnel file, Theodore B. Hayne, RAC.

46. Hayne to Fannie Thorn Hayne, July 12, 1929. WHL.

47. Hayne to Fannie Thorn Hayne, April 25, 1929. WHL.

48. Hayne to Fannie Thorn Hayne, June 19, 1929. WHL.

49. Hayne to Fannie Thorn Hayne, July 12, 1929. WHL.

50. The Rockefeller Foundation. *Annual Report, 1930* (New York: The Rockefeller Foundation, 1930), 34. These data were reported in the literature after Hayne's death. See: Henry Beeuwkes, J. H. Bauer, A. F. Mahaffy, "Yellow Fever Endemicity in West Africa, with Special Reference to Protection Tests," *American Journal of Tropical Medicine* 10 (1930): 305-333.

51. "Report on Ibadan Area," in: Fifth Annual Report, West African Yellow Fever Commission, 1929. RAC.

52. At that time, statistical analysis of data was not commonly carried out. These results, however, do not quite achieve statistical significance (p–0.056 by chi-square test).

53. Diary—Henry Beeuwkes, December 24, 1929, RAC.

54. The Rockefeller Foundation, *Annual Report, 1930* (New York: The Rockefeller Foundation, 1930), 31.

55. Ibid, 32.

56. *Mansonia africana* was then known as *Taeniorhynchus (Mansonioides) africanus*. Although this mosquito is highly prevalent in West Africa and can transmit the yellow fever virus in the laboratory, the virus has never been found in wild-caught specimens.

57. Barber, *A Malariologist in Many Lands*, 69.

58. Hayne to Fannie Thorn Hayne, March 11, 1929. WHL.

59. Hayne to Frances Thorn Hayne, July 12, 1929. WHL. Hayne's pes-

simism that nobody noted or cared about this work was not entirely correct. The annual report of the West African Yellow Fever Commission observed that between 70% and 100% of the school children in Abeokuta, Ife, and Ibadan carried malaria parasites. It was also mentioned that Hayne found malaria in 25 Nigerian boy scouts at the Ibadan Training College. An identical percentage of students and laborers at the Training College had malaria parasites.

60. Hayne to Fannie Thorn Hayne, November 13, 1928. WHL.

61. Hayne to Fannie Thorn Hayne, June 30, 1929. WHL.

62. Hayne to Fannie Thorn Hayne, July 12, 1929. WHL.

63. Ibid.

64. Diary—Henry Beeuwkes, September 20, 1929, RAC.

65. Thomas H. G. Aitken, "Henry William Kumm, 1901-1991," *Journal of the American Mosquito Control Association* 7 (1991): 673-674.

66. J. S. Porterfield, "Yellow fever in West Africa: A Retrospective Glance," *British Medical Journal* 299 (1989): 1555-1557. Porterfield briefly mentions Hayne as "Edward Haynes."

67. Diary—Henry Beeuwkes, October 3, 1929, RAC.

68. Diary—Henry Beeuwkes, November 5, 1929, RAC.

69. Diary—Henry Beeuwkes, November 16, 1929, RAC.

70. Diary—Henry Beeuwkes, November 20, 1929, RAC.

71. Hayne to Fannie Thorn Hayne, November 17, 1929. WHL.

72. Diary—Henry Beeuwkes, November 16, 1929, RAC.

73. Diary—Henry Beeuwkes, October 16, 1929, RAC.

74. Beeuwkes to Russell, October 12, 1929. Personnel file, Theodore B. Hayne, RAC.

75. Hayne to Lillah Adams Hayne, October 7, 1928. WHL.

76. Hayne to Philip Gadsden Hasell, November 2, 1928.

77. Hayne to Fannie Thorn Hayne, June 19, 1929. WHL.

78. James Adams Hayne, "The History of Pellagra in South Carolina," *Journal of the South Carolina Medical Association*, 28 (1932): 205-209. Pellagra was recognized in South Carolina during the early 1900s, but its cause had sparked great controversy. Some blamed insects; others blamed bodily excretions and poor hygiene; while still others blamed diet. Joseph Goldberger and his colleagues with the United States Public Health Service determined that pellagra is due to dietary deficiency. Some of the crucial experiments were carried out in South Carolina. Dried Brewer's yeast was found to be effective therapy. Under Adams Hayne's supervision, the South Carolina State Board of Health began to distribute Brewer's yeast by

the ton. The number of deaths attributed to pellagra fell from 1,306 in 1915 and to 219 by 1920. However, the boll weevil, deflation, and economic depression brought it out again, and the number had climbed to 927 deaths in 1928. Hence, the problem of pellagra was still not resolved.

79. James A. Hayne, "Endemic Goiter and Its Relation to Iodine Content of Food," *American Journal of Public Health* 19 (1929): 1111-1118. In 1895, it was determined that the thyroid gland contains an organic compound of iodine. Later, it was realized that goiter—often caused by lack of iodine—was uncommon in South Carolina. This observation was in turn attributed to the high iodine content of the state's soil, and therefore of its fruits and vegetables. Adams Hayne reasoned that fruits and vegetables with high iodine content would be superior to the pure mineral (as contained in iodized salt). He made an analogy to pernicious anemia, in which it had been found that whole liver extract was therapeutic whereas copper, manganese, and iron salts were not. However, the analogy was later found to be incorrect: Pernicious anemia is caused by deficiency of vitamin B12, which just happened to be contained in the liver extract. Just as the bone marrow requires only vitamin B12, so does the thyroid require only elemental iodine. Hence, there was nothing special about the iodine contained in fruits and vegetables. At the 44th Annual Conference of State and Provincial Health Authorities of North America, Adams Hayne proclaimed: "We know that South Carolina fruits and vegetables contain sufficient iodine for nutritional purposes, and if people will eat South Carolina fruits and vegetables they may reasonably expect not to have goiter." It is telling that in his letter to his son, he confesses that this idea might be "a castle in Spain."

80. Hayne to Fannie Thorn Hayne, July 12, 1929. WHL.

81. James Adams Hayne to Theodore Brevard Hayne, November 5, 1929. WHL.

82. Hayne to Fannie Thorn Hayne, November 17, 1929. WHL.

83. Diary—Henry Beeuwkes, December 5, 1929, RAC.

84. Fifth Annual Report, West African Yellow Fever Commission, 1929. RAC. Hayne drew blood for protection tests from 34 children between the ages of four and ten. The data were considered to be important because Sierra Leone had once been a hotbed of yellow fever, but no cases had been confirmed since 1919. Was the disease endemic there?

85. Diary—Henry Beeuwkes, December 31, 1929, RAC.

86. Russell to Hayne. Personnel file, Theodore B. Hayne, RAC.

5. Diagnosis Yellow Fever

1. Confidential Report of Medical Examiner, January 2, 1929 [1930, see p. 85]. Personnel file, Theodore B. Hayne, RAC.
2. Hayne to Fannie Thorn Hayne, April 3, 1930. WHL.
3. Henry W. Kumm to Hayne, March 16, 1930. WHL.
4. Hayne to James Adams Hayne, April 3, 1930. WHL.
5. Ibid.
6. Hayne to Fannie Thorn Hayne, April 14, 1930. WHL.
7. Hayne to Fannie Thorn Hayne, April 3, 1930. WHL.
8. Barber to Russell, March 10, 1929. Personnel file, Marshall A. Barber. RAC.
9. Excerpt from Henry Beeuwkes' diary, January 21, 1930. Personnel file, Theodore B. Hayne, RAC.
10. Technically, W. A. Young was a British investigator not employed by the Rockefeller Foundation. However, he is included among the Rockefeller Foundation yellow fever casualties in the standard accounts of this period because his death was attributed to assisting Noguchi with research carried out under Rockefeller auspices. The Rockefeller Foundation paid an allowance to Young's family.
11. The Rockefeller Foundation, *Annual Report, 1929* (New York: The Rockefeller Foundation, 1929), 50-51.
12. Russell to Beeuwkes, June 20, 1930. Personnel file, Marshall A. Barber. RAC.
13. These mosquitoes were classified into three groups, as follows: (1) "Mansonioides", later found to include two species: *Taeniorhynchus (M.) africanus* and *T. (M.) uniformis*; (2) tree-hole breeding mosquitoes, which included *Aedes africanus*, Theo.; *Aedes luteocephalus*, Newst., *Aedes stokesi*, Evans, *Aedes simpsoni*, Theo., and occasionally *Eretmodites chrysogaster*, Graham; and (3) *Aedes irritans*, Theo., and *Aedes nigricephalus*, Theo.
14. Diary—Henry Beeuwkes, May 2, 1930, RAC.
15. Diary—Henry Beeuwkes, May 30, 1930, RAC.
16. Hayne to Fannie Thorn Hayne, June 15, 1930. WHL.
17. J. A. Kerr, "Report of the Work of the Entomology Laboratory," in Sixth Annual Report, West African Yellow Fever Commission, 1930. RAC.
18. J. A. Kerr to Fannie Thorn Hayne, December 28, 1930. WHL.
19. Diary—Henry Beeuwkes, June 10, 1930, RAC.
20. Kerr, "Report of the Work of the Entomology Laboratory."
21. Barber jested in his autobiography:

It occurs to me that an outdoor African audience might be useful for a preview of certain kinds of movie (just as it was once customary to exhibit a legitimate play to a college audience before taking it to New York). If the people never squirm, however severely bitten, the film might be considered a success and immediately transported to New York and exhibited there (Barber, *A Malariologist in Many Lands*, 70–71).

22. Diary—Henry Beeuwkes, May 10, 1930, RAC.
23. Ibid.
24. Diary—Henry Beeuwkes, June 16, 1930, RAC.
25. Barber, *A Malariologist in Many Lands*, 73.
26. Kerr, "Report of the Work of the Entomology Laboratory."
27. Hayne to Isaac Hayne, June 22, 1930. WHL.
28. J. A. Kerr, "Report of the Work of the Entomology Laboratory."
29. Diary—Henry Beeuwkes, June 16, 1930, RAC.
30. Diary—Henry Beeuwkes, May 22, 1930, RAC.
31. Ibid.
32. Diary—Henry Beeuwkes, May 24, 1930, RAC.
33. Hayne to unidentified recipient [probably Isaac Hayne], undated. WHL
34. Diary—Henry Beeuwkes, August 23, 1930, RAC.
35. Diary—Henry Beeuwkes, June 12, 1930, RAC.
36. Diary—Henry Beeuwkes, June 10, 1930, RAC.
37. Ibid.
38. Hayne to Fannie Thorn Hayne, June 15, 1930. WHL.
39. Ibid.
40. Hayne to Isaac Hayne, June 22, 1930. WHL.
41. Nadine M. Barber to Fannie Thorn Hayne, August 16, 1930. WHL.
42. Hayne to Isaac Hayne, June 22, 1930. WHL.
43. Ibid.
44. Ibid.
45. Hayne to Fannie Thorn Hayne, June 21-22, 1930. WHL.
46. Fannie Thorn Hayne to Hayne, June 24, 1930. WHL.
47. Hayne to Fannie Thorn Hayne, June 15, 1930. WHL.
48. Fannie Thorn Hayne to Hayne, July 5, 1930. WHL.
49. History on the case of Dr. T. B. Hayne, American, 31 years of age, in charge of the Entomological Laboratory of the West African Yellow Fever Commission, Lagos, Nigeria. Personnel file, Theodore B. Hayne, RAC.

50. Diary—Henry Beeuwkes, July 8, 1930, RAC.
51. Fannie Thorn Hayne to Hayne, July 8, 1930. WHL.
52. Diary—Henry Beeuwkes, July 8, 1930, RAC.
53. Ibid.
54. History on the case of Dr. T. B. Hayne, American. Personnel file, Theodore B. Hayne, RAC.
55. Diary—Henry Beeuwkes, July 9, 1930, RAC.
56. Ibid.
57. Diary—Henry Beeuwkes, July 10, 1930, RAC.
58. Ibid.
59. Ibid.
60. Beeuwkes to Rockefeller Foundation, July 30, 1930. Personnel file, Theodore B. Hayne, RAC.
61. Diary—Henry Beeuwkes, July 10, 1930, RAC.
62. History on the case of Dr. T. B. Hayne, American. Personnel file, Theodore B. Hayne, RAC.
63. Diary—Henry Beeuwkes, July 10, 1930, RAC.
64. The Rockefeller Foundation. *Annual Report, 1930* (New York: The Rockefeller Foundation, 1930), 38.
65. Diary—Henry Beeuwkes, July 11, 1930, RAC.
66. Beeuwkes to Russell, July 18, 1930. Personnel file, Theodore B. Hayne, RAC.
67. Diary—Henry Beeuwkes, July 12, 1930, RAC.
68. N. Paul Hudson, "Microscopic examination of tissues of Dr. T. B. Hayne," November 18, 1930. Personnel file, Theodore B. Hayne, RAC.
69. Oskar Klotz [review of microscopic sections of the case of Dr. T. B. Hayne]. Personnel file, Theodore B. Hayne, RAC.
70. O. Klotz to Russell, August 20, 1930. Personnel file, Theodore B. Hayne, RAC.
71. S. Kitchen to Russell, August 20, 1930. Personnel file, Theodore B. Hayne, RAC.
72. Fred L. Soper to Russell, September 10, 1930. Personnel file, Theodore B. Hayne, RAC.
73. Russell to Beeuwkes, July 24, 1930. Personnel file, Theodore B. Hayne, RAC.
74. Russell to H. T. Chickering, August 25, 1930. Personnel file, Theodore B. Hayne, RAC.
75. The Rockefeller Foundation. *Annual Report, 1930* (New York: The Rockefeller Foundation, 1930), 60.

76. Nelson C. Davis, "Attempts to Determine the Amount of Yellow Fever Virus Injected by the Bite of a Single Stegomyia Mosquito," *American Journal of Tropical Medicine* 14 (1934): 343-354.

77. Johannes H. Bauer, "Some Characteristics of Yellow Fever Virus," *American Journal of Tropical Medicine* 11 (1931): 337-353.

78. See G. P. Berry and S. F. Kitchen, "Yellow Fever Accidentally Acquired in the Laboratory," *American Journal of Tropical Medicine* 11 (1931): 365-434. Hayne's case (number 27) was attributed to the "bite of infective mosquito."

79. Diary—Henry Beeuwkes, July 21, 1930. RAC. For confirmation of Wright's identity, see *Crockford's Clerical Directory for 1930* (59th ed., London: Oxford University Press, 1930), 1456.

80. Diary—Henry Beeuwkes, July 12, 1930, RAC.

81. Beeuwkes to Russell, July 17, 1930. Personnel file, Theodore B. Hayne, RAC.

6. Coming Home

1. H. H. Scott to Beeuwkes, August 12, 1930. Personnel file, Theodore B. Hayne, RAC.

2. W. B. Johnson to Beeuwkes, July 14, 1930. Personnel file, Theodore B. Hayne, RAC.

3. Cyril Truelove to Beeuwkes, July 11, 1930. Personnel file, Theodore B. Hayne, RAC.

4. H. B. Lee to Beeuwkes, July 11, 1930. Personnel file, Theodore B. Hayne, RAC.

5. Burial of Dr. Theodore B. Hayne: diary of George H. Ramsey. Personnel file, Theodore B. Hayne, RAC.

6. Ibid. Actually, Swanson Lunsford, who served as a captain in Lee's Legion during the American Revolution, died in Columbia, S.C. on August 7, 1799. See *South Carolina Historical and Genealogical Magazine* 8 (1907): 221-222.

7. Ibid.

8. Ibid.

9. Ibid.

10. The order of service survives: The Exhortation; Hymn 197; Wisdom 3: 1-9; Psalm 23; 2 Corinthians 5: 1-10; Hymn 140; Prayers; The Blessing; The Nunc dimittis; The Dead March.

11. Burial of Dr. Theodore B. Hayne: diary of George H. Ramsey. Personnel file, Theodore B. Hayne, RAC.

12. Fred L. Soper to James A. Hayne, July 25, 1930. Personnel file, Theodore B. Hayne, RAC.

13. O. Klotz to Russell, August 20, 1930. Personnel file, Theodore B. Hayne, RAC.

14. Sixth Annual Report, West African Yellow Fever Commission, 1930. RAC.

15. W. H. Frost to Russell, December 8, 1930. Personnel file, Theodore B. Hayne, RAC.

16. Dr. Hayne—Resolution Upon Death. Personnel file, Theodore B. Hayne, RAC.

17. Nadine M. Barber to Dr. and Mrs. James Adams Hayne, July 19, 1930. WHL.

18. Nadine M. Barber to Fannie Thorn Hayne, August 16, 1930. WHL

19. J. A. Kerr to Fannie Thorn Hayne, December 28, 1930. WHL.

20. Kerr, "Report of the Work of the Entomology Laboratory," in Sixth Annual Report, West African Yellow Fever Commission, 1930. RAC.

21. Kerr, "Studies on the Abundance, Distribution and Feeding Habits of Some West African Mosquitoes," *Bulletin of Entomological Research* 24 (1933): 493-510.

22. J. A. Kerr and T. B. Hayne, "On the Transfer of Yellow Fever Virus from Female to Male Aedes Aegypti," *American Journal of Tropical Medicine* 12 (1932): 255-261.

23. Henry Beeuwkes and T. B. Hayne, "An Experimental Demonstration of the Infectivity with Yellow Fever Virus of *Aedes aegypti* Captured in an African Town," *Transactions of the Royal Society of Tropical Medicine and Hygiene* 25 (1931): 107-110.

24. The Rockefeller Foundation. *Annual Report, 1930* (New York: The Rockefeller Foundation, 1931).

Epilogue: "That's Theodore's Car"

1. Roselle Hayne to Russell, November 28, 1930. Personnel file, Theodore B. Hayne, RAC.

2. Max Theiler, "Susceptiblity of White Mice to the Virus of Yellow Fever," *Science* 71 (April 4, 1930): 367.

3. The Rockefeller Foundation. *Annual Report, 1930* (New York: The Rockefeller Foundation, 1930), 44.

4. W. A. Sawyer, S. F. Kitchen, and W. Lloyd, "Vaccination of Humans Against Yellow Fever with Immune Serum and Virus Fixed for Mice,"

Proceedings of the Society for Experimental Biology and Medicine 29 (1931): 62-64.

5. The Rockefeller Foundation. *Annual Report, 1931* (New York: The Rockefeller Foundation, 1931), 35.

6. F. L. Soper, H. A. Penna, E. Cardoso, J. Serafim, Jr., M. Frobisher, Jr., and J. Pinheiro: "Yellow Fever Without *Aedes aegypti:* Study of Rural Epidemic in Valle do Chanaan, Espirito Santo, Brazil, 1932, *American Journal of Hygiene* 18 (1932): 555-587.

7. The Rockefeller Foundation. *Annual Report, 1934* (New York: The Rockefeller Foundation, 1934), 7.

8. Wesley W. Spink, *Infectious Diseases: Prevention and Treatment in the Nineteenth and Twentieth Centuries* (Minneapolis: University of Minnesota Press, 1978), 158.

9. A. Nasidi, T. P. Monath, K. DeCock, et al., "Urban Yellow Fever Epidemic in Western Nigeria, 1987," *Transactions of the Royal Society of Tropical Medicine and Hygiene* 83 (1989): 401-406.

10. Thomas P. Monath, "Yellow Fever: A Medically Neglected Disease. Report on a Seminar." *Reviews of Infectious Diseases* 9 (1987): 163-175.

11. P. L. J. Brès, "A Century of Progress in Combatting Yellow Fever," *Bulletin of the World Health Organization* 64 (1986): 775-786.

12. Laura Jervey Hopkins, personal communication.

Index

Abeokuta, Nigeria, 61, 62, 72
Accra, Gold Coast [Ghana], 49, 52
Adams, Elizabeth ("Lillah")
    See Hayne, Elizabeth Adams
    ("Lillah," 1850-1937)
Aedes aegypti mosquito, 9-10, 13, 37, 44-
    46, 48, 51, 53, 72, 76-77, 88-90, 92-
    96, 124-125, 128
Aedes africanus mosquito, 89, 92
Aedes apicoannulatus mosquito, 53
Aedes apicoargenteus mosquito, 89
Aedes costalis mosquito, 123
Aedes irritans mosquito, 89, 90, 92, 105
Aedes longipalpis mosquito, 89
Aedes luteocephalus mosquito, 53, 89, 92
Aedes nigricephalus mosquito, 89, 90
Aedes occidentalis mosquito
See Aedes stokesi
Aedes stokesi mosquito, 89, 90, 92, 125
Aedes vittatus (sugens) mosquito, 72
Africa, continent of, 43, 81-82, 104-
    105, 129.
    See also specific countries; West Af-
    rica
AIDS epidemic, 2-4
Alabama, 1, 44
Ali (Nigerian), 110
Amazon Valley, 128-129
American Revolution, 8, 10, 116,
    155n.6
Ancon, Canal Zone, 36, 38, 86
Ancon Hospital
    See Gorgas Hospital
Anopheles mosquitoes, 8, 10, 19-24, 30-
    33, 46, 77, 88, 95, 105
Anopheles crucians, 20

Anopheles punctipennis, 20-21
Anopheles quadrimaculatus, 20-21, 35
Arkansas, State of, 29, 33, 35, 90
Army, United States
    See United States Army
Asbestos Company of Philadelphia, 49
Ascariasis, 100
Asibi (Nigerian), 50-51, 54
Athens, Georgia, 11
Atlanta, Georgia, 8
Auchi, Brazil, 56

Bahia, Brazil, 87, 97
Baltimore, Maryland, 43, 86, 103
Banov, Leon, 116-117
Barber, Marshall Albert, 28-33, 35-36,
    39, 60, 74-75, 77-78, 87, 88, 90, 94-
    95, 98-99, 102, 106, 120-121, 130
Barber, Nadine, 87, 97, 98, 102, 112,
    120-122
Bartonellosis, 1
Bassett, John Y., 1
Bauer, Johannes, 51, 53, 76, 77, 87, 111
Baynard, R. S. ("Bud"), 26
Beattie, Hamlin ("Ham"), 17, 68, 87, 97,
    117
Beeuwkes, Henry, 1, 4, 40, 48-52, 55,
    58-60, 62-66, 68-69, 71, 75-78, 83,
    87-97, 102, 104-113, 115, 119, 123,
    125-126, 129
Blackstock, South Carolina, 3, 11, 12
Bolivia, 43, 129
Bond, O. J., 26
Boston, Massachusetts, 1, 43
Bottineau, North Dakota, 31
Boyce, Rupert, 72

Brazil, 44, 49, 87, 119, 128-129
Brewton, Alabama, 33
Burke, A. W., 91, 93, 94, 97, 106, 109

Calcutta, India, 8
Camilla, Georgia, 31
Camp Columbia, Cuba, 9
Camp Jackson [Fort Jackson], South
    Carolina, 28
Carnegie, Andrew, 45
Carrión, Daniel A., 1
Carter, Henry Rose, 8-10, 13, 15, 19-
    22, 27, 34, 39, 40, 46-47,55, 120
Carter, Laura, 20, 40-41, 55, 119
Cat Island, Mississippi, 33
Catawba River, 21-22
Centers for Disease Control, 2
Chamberlain, Dorothy, 16
Charleston, South Carolina, 10, 17, 24,
    33, 34, 44, 98, 116-117,119
Chester, South Carolina, 11
Chester County, South Carolina, 21
Cheyenne, Wyoming, 17
Chicago, Illinois, 17, 90
Chickering, H. T., 85, 111
Cholera, 1
Citadel, The, 11, 24-28, 34
Civil War, American, 10-11, 24
Colleton Cypress Company, The, 22-
    24
Colombia, 129
Colonial Medical Research Committee,
    115
Columbia, South Carolina, 7, 14, 33, 44,
    65, 85, 97, 102-103,116-118, 127
Columbia (South Carolina) Medical
    Society, 3, 5
Congaree, South Carolina, 2, 17, 28, 65,
    78, 85, 97, 101-102,104, 115, 117-
    118, 127
Costa Rica, 39
Craig, Sarah, 12

Cross, Howard B., 48, 112
Cuba, 44, 46
Culex decens mosquitoes, 95
Culex duttoni mosquitoes, 95
Culex nebulosus mosquitoes, 95

Dakar, French Equatorial Africa
    [Senegal], 49
Darling, Samuel Taylor, 41
Davis, George Wilmot, 79
Davis, Gordon, 63
DDT, 32
Dengue fever, 62
Douglas, Davison M., 118
Douglas, Jan, 14
Dublin, Ireland, 50

Ecuador, 46-47
Eddu, Nigeria, 88
Ede, Nigeria, 65
El Cajon, California, 130
El Salvador, country of, 49
Ellenton, South Carolina, 98
England, 73, 83, 86, 101
    colonists in North America, 7
    customs of, 57-88
Eretmapoditis chrysogaster mosquito, 53
Euba Metta, Nigeria, 57
European Hospital, Lagos, 51, 66-67,
    106-108
Exchange Building, Charleston, 10

Ferrell, John A., 39-40
Fiji Islands, 29
Filariasis, 73
Finlay, Carlos J., 9-10
Fort Assiniboine, Montana, 15-16
Fort D. A. Russell, Montana, 17
Fort Jackson, South Carolina
    See Camp Jackson
Fort Lawn, South Carolina, 21
Fort Sumter, South Carolina, 11, 24

Freetown, Sierra Leone, 82-83
French Canal Company, 36
Frost, Wade Hampton, 119-120
Furman College, 11

Glasounoff, Vladimir, 57, 89, 91, 93, 94, 95
Goiter, 82
Gold Coast [Ghana], 108
Gorgas, William Crawford, 10, 13, 15, 37, 44-47
Gorgas Hospital, Ancon, Canal Zone, 36-39, 41, 86
Gorgas Memorial Research Laboratory, 74
Gray, Dr., 106-108
Greenville, South Carolina, 11, 14
Guatemala, 49
Guayaquil, Ecuador, 46-47
Guinea worm, 100
Guy's Hospital, London, 50

Hamburg, Germany, 50
Harvard University, 1
Hasell, Frances Hayne
  See Hayne, Frances Thorn ("Frank")
Hasell, Philip Gadsden ("Shrimp"), 6, 17, 24-26, 34-35, 56, 58, 62, 68, 78, 98, 101, 117-118, 130
Hasell, Philip Gadsden, Jr. ("Toli"), 105
Hasell family, 34
Havana, Cuba, 7, 9
Hayne, Adams
  See James Adams Hayne (1872-1953)
Hayne, Alicia Shubrick, 12
Hayne, Elizabeth Adams ("Lillah," 1850-1937), 11, 117, 139 n.25
Hayne, Fannie Douglass ("Fan"), 3, 6, 11, 34-35, 38, 65-66, 69, 73-74, 86-88, 90, 97-98, 101-105, 120-125, 130

Hayne, Frances Thorn ("Frank"; later, Frances Thorn Hasell), 6, 12, 13, 25, 26, 34, 98
Hayne, Isaac (1745-1781), 10, 67
Hayne, Isaac ("Ike") (1906-1974), 6, 12, 16, 34, 40, 62-63, 94, 98-101, 116, 130
Hayne, James Adams (1872-1953), 3, 5-7, 11-17, 19-22, 27, 33, 38, 65, 68, 78-82, 85-86, 102-103, 116, 120-121, 130
  as state health officer, 17, 20-21, 27, 79-82, 130
  character, 11-12
  in Spanish-American War, 7, 11
  "The Rights of the Child," 11-12
Hayne, James Adams II ("The Doctor," 1911-1983), 6, 12, 98, 130
Hayne, Lillah Adams (1902-1992), 12, 13, 57, 61, 78, 98, 104
Hayne, Margaret Johnson ("Daisy"), 12, 104
Hayne, Mary Lunsford, 12, 16, 79, 81, 87
Hayne, Paul Hamilton, 10
Hayne, Robert Young, 10
Hayne, Roselle Hundley, 6, 38-39, 78, 81, 85, 87, 97-99, 101-105, 112, 117-118, 127, 130
Hayne, Susan Wilhelmina, 12, 79, 87
Hayne, Susie Stevenson, 130
Hayne, Theodore Brevard (1841-1917), 10-11
Hayne, Theodore Brevard, Jr. (1878-1878), 135n.23
Hayne, Theodore Brevard (1898-1930), 2-6, 7, 10-18, 19-41, 54, 55-83, 85-113, 115-126, 127, 130
  automobiles and, 17, 34-35, 36, 59, 62, 65, 66-68, 85, 130
  birth of, 3, 7, 10, 12
  childhood and youth, 11-18

Hayne, Theodore Brevard (cont.)
  in college, 24-28
  death of, 102-108
  eulogies of, 3, 112, 115-116, 119-120
  in flight school, 25-26
  funeral of, 118
  health of, 31, 55, 66-68, 85, 95
  malaria investigations of, 19-24, 28-33, 35-36, 40-41, 73
  marriage of, 85-86
  in medical school, 33-36
  memorial service for, 112
  in Nigeria, 55-83, 86-113
  in Panama, 15, 36-41
  Paris green, investigations of, 31-33
  personality of, 4-5, 12, 18, 24-25, 27, 59, 68, 83, 115,119-123
  post-mortem examination of, 108-112
  yellow fever investigations of, 59-65, 69-78, 82-83, 87-101,104-105, 119-126
Hayne, Theodore Brevard IV (1953-), 4, 130
Hayne family, 10, 34, 127, 130
Hayne-Webster debate, 10
Hookworm, 29, 45, 100
Hudson, Paul, 51, 110
Human immunodeficiency virus
  See AIDS epidemic
Hundley, Anne Roselle
  See Hayne, Roselle Hundley

Ibadan, Nigeria, 49, 56, 59-61, 64, 69-70, 72-73, 75, 95-97, 100,104, 115
Ibadan District, Nigeria, 59-60, 69, 71, 75
Ife, Nigeria, 56, 64, 70, 76
Ijebu Ode, Nigeria, 61, 67, 70
Ilorin, Nigeria, 70
India, 130
Influenza, 26, 57, 62, 106

International Health Board
  See Rockefeller Foundation, International Health Board
Iodine, 79, 82
Isthmian Canal Service, 13-15
Iwonran, Nigeria, 88, 91, 93

Jackson, James, Jr., 1
Johns Hopkins University and Medical Institutions, 48, 49, 56,87, 103, 129
Jos, Nigeria, 70, 71
Journal of the American Medical Association, 11
Journal of the South Carolina Medical Association, 4

Kano, Nigeria, 71
Kansas, 29
Kerr, John Austin, 5, 90, 91, 97, 106, 123-125, 130
Key center theory, 46-47
Kitchen, S. F., 110-111
Klotz, Oskar, 59, 110, 119
Kukuruku disease, 65
Kumm, Henry W., 5, 56, 59, 63, 75, 85-86, 116-118, 130

Lagos, Nigeria, 3, 4, 41, 48-49, 51, 55-57, 64-67, 72, 74, 78,82, 86, 90, 97-99, 106, 112-113, 115, 117-118, 122
Lake, Kirsopp, 1
Lake Murray, South Carolina, 86, 118
Larteh, Gold Coast [Ghana], 50
Lazear, Jesse, 1-2, 9
Le Prince, Joseph Augustin, 13-15, 19-22, 92, 120
Leptospira icteroides, 46-50
Leptospirosis, 46, 62
de Lesseps, Ferdinand, 13
Lewis, Paul, 87, 112
Liberia, 64
Little Salkehatchie Swamp, 22-24

Liverpool, England, 55
Liverpool School of Tropical Medicine, 129
London, England, 47, 50, 115
Louisiana, 35
Louisiana Territory, 7
Louisville, Kentucky, 68
Lunsford, Swanson, 116, 155 (note 6)
Lynchburg, Virginia, 117

MacDougall, Dr., 83
Mackey, Dr., 67
Mahaffy, A. F., 50, 67, 101-102, 105
Malaria, 7-8, 10, 13, 15, 19-24, 26, 28-33, 35-36, 40-41, 57, 59, 62, 64, 67, 72-74, 81, 88, 95, 99-100, 106, 120, 130
    control projects, 20-21
    history of, 7-8
    mosquitoes in transmission of, 8, 13, 19-24, 26, 28-33, 35-36
    See also Anopheles mosquitoes; Hayne, Theodore Brevard(1898-1930), malaria investigations of

Malaya [Malay Peninsula], 29, 45
Malta fever, 62
Mansonia africana mosquito, 72
"Mansonioides" mosquitoes, 95-96, 105
Munsonioides africanus mosquito, 90, 92, 96
Mason, Max, 1
Medical College of the State of South Carolina, 11, 33-36
Memphis, Tennessee, 28, 29, 44
Mississippi, 9, 33, 35-36
Mobile, Alabama, 44
Monrovia, Liberian Republic, 64, 102
Montana, 15-17
Mosquitoes, 2, 4-5, 7-10, 13-15, 19-24, 29-33, 35-37, 47-48, 51-54, 56, 58, 64, 67, 70, 72, 75-77, 85, 93-98, 105, 109-111, 123-125

Mosquitoes (cont.)
    control of, 13-15, 19-21, 29-33, 35-36, 44, 53-54
    flight experiments with, 21-22, 92-94
    "night catches with human bait," 29-31, 90-92
    tree-hole and crab-hole breeding, 87-92
    See also individual species; malaria; Paris green
Mount Pleasant, South Carolina, 34

Napoleon Bonaparte, 7
Nashville, Tennessee, 45
Naval Aviation School, 25-26
Navy, United States
    See United States Navy
Newberry, South Carolina, 16
New Orleans, Louisiana, 12, 32, 44
New York, New York, 36, 43, 46, 50, 54-55, 82-83, 85-87, 107, 113, 119-120
Newton, Pennsylvania, 130
Nigeria, 3-5, 48-54, 86, 88, 100, 108, 129
    See also specific cities and towns; Hayne, Theodore Brevard(1898-1930), in Nigeria; West Africa
Nile River, 128
Noguchi, Hideyo, 46-48, 51-52, 112
North Augusta, South Carolina, 21
Nott, Josiah Clark, 44

Odumyao, Nigeria, 88
Ogbomosho, Nigeria, 59
Onitiri, Nigeria, 88
Orangeburg, South Carolina, 81
Oshogbo, Nigeria, 64-65, 70
Osler, William, 1, 8
Ossining, New York, 130
Otta, Nigeria, 92-94
Oyo, Nigeria, 61, 70

Panama, 13-15, 36-40, 44-46, 57, 85
Panama Canal, 13, 19, 45
Panama Canal Commission, 15
Paris, France, 1, 78, 82
Paris green, 31-33
Peabody, Francis Weld, 1
Pellagra, 79
Pershing, John J., 49
Peru, 129
Philadelphia, Pennsylvania, 43
Philip, C. B. ("Neil"), 5, 56, 63, 74-75, 78, 130
Phillipines, 29, 45
Phillips, W. F. R., 34
Plague, 56, 99-100
Pneumonia, 64
Pocantico Hills, New York, 4
Poliomyelitis, 87
Ponjuponju, 65
Porter, Anthony Toomer, 17
Porter Military Academy, 17
Protection tests, 69-72, 96-97, 127-128
Public Health Service, United States
    See United States Public Health Service

Ramsey, George H., 116-118
Reed, Walter, 9, 21, 44
Reed Commission, 9-10, 44
Relapsing fever, 62, 64, 65, 73
Revolutionary War
    See American Revolution
Ricketts, Howard Taylor, 2
"Rights of the Child, The," 11-12
Rio de Janeiro, Brazil, 101
Rockefeller, John D., 45
Rockefeller, John D., Jr., 1
Rockefeller Archive Center, 4
Rockefeller Foundation, 4, 39-41, 43-54, 55, 57, 60-61, 65, 68,72, 74, 83, 87, 98, 100-101, 103, 107-108, 111-112, 116, 119,125-126, 127-130

Rockefeller Foundation (cont.)
    history of, 45
    International Health Board (Division), 1, 39-41, 45-54, 55-83, 111
    West African Yellow Fever Commission, 43, 48-54, 55-83, 119,121-122, 124-125
Rockefeller Institute for Medical Research, 46
Rocky Mountain spotted fever, 130
Rose, Wickliffe, 45
Ross, Ronald, 8, 10
Rush, Benjamin, 43-44
Russell, Frederick F., 41, 55, 58, 68, 78, 83, 86-88, 109-111,113, 116, 119
Russia, 49

San Diego, California, 25, 117
San Francisco, California, 130
Sawyer, Wilbur A., 49, 54, 129
Schistosomiasis, 73, 100
Seattle, Washington, 25-26
Senegal, 128
Ship Island, Missisippi, 33
Sierra Leone, 82-83
Sleeping sickness, 100
Smith, Hugh H., 129
Soper, Fred L., 111, 119
South America, 94, 99, 100, 101, 129
    See also specific countries
South Carolina, 6, 15-17, 22, 73, 79-82, 87, 130
    economy of, 79, 81-82
    public health of, 5-6, 17, 79, 80-82
South Carolina Medical Association, 118
South Caroliniana Library, 3
Southern Medical Journal, 36
Spain, colonists in North America, 7
Spanish-American War, 7, 9, 11, 103
Stegomyia
    See *Aedes aegypti*

Sternberg, George, 9
Stokes, Adrian, 50-52, 112, 118, 121, 125
Stuttgart, Arkansas, 29-31
Suez Canal, 13
Syphilis, 46

Taboga Island, Panama, 14, 38
Taeniorhynchus africanus mosquito
See *Mansonioides africanus*
Tapeworm, 100
Theiler, Max, 127, 129
Thorn, Adalize, 11, 16
Thorn, Fannie Douglass
See Hayne, Fannie Thorn
Toronto, Canada, 119
Treponema pallidum, 46
Tuberculosis, 20, 109
Tuxtepec, Mexico, 48
Typhoid fever, 19
Typhus, 2

United States Army, 7, 15
United States Navy, 25-26
United States Public Health Service, 8-9, 20, 28-33, 74, 120
University of Chicago, 110
University of Kansas, 29
University of Nebraska, 56
University of South Carolina, 11, 118
University of Toronto, 110
University of Virginia, 11

Vera Cruz, Mexico, 48
Vicksburg, Mississipi, 44

Walcott, A. M., 56, 96
Washington, District of Columbia, 11, 26, 28, 31, 82, 86
Water hyacinth, 35
Wavering Place, 15, 17-18, 32, 79, 80, 85, 97, 117-118, 130

Weathersbee, Albert Allen, 98
Weil's disease
See Leptospirosis
West Africa, 3-4, 19, 21, 29, 40-41, 47-54, 59, 64, 69, 71-72, 74-75, 85, 88, 99, 120, 128
See also specific localities and Rockefeller Foundation, West African Yellow Fever Commission
West African Yellow Fever Commission
See Rockefeller Foundation, West African Yellow Fever Commission
Williams, G. Croft, 118
Williams, Louis L., 119
World War I, 25, 28, 56
World War II, 130
Wright, Ruthven Alexanderson, 112

Yaba, Nigeria, 4-5, 41, 49, 55-59, 61, 87-88, 92, 98, 103, 108, 110, 120, 123, 125, 129
See also Rockefeller Foundation, West African Yellow Fever Commission
Yaws, 100
Yellow fever, 1-5, 7-10, 13, 15, 17, 24, 37, 40-41, 43-54, 56, 60-65, 69-73, 75, 77, 86-88, 95-101, 104-112, 116, 120-126, 127-130
history of, 7-10, 43-54
jungle yellow fever, 44-45
pathology and pathogenesis of, 44-45
role of mosquitoes other than *A. aegypti* in transmission of, 44, 53, 72, 88-92, 124-125, 128-129
urban yellow fever, 44-45
See also *Aedes* aegypti; flight experiments; key center theory; "night catches with human bait"; protection tests; Rockefeller Founda-

Yellow fever (cont.)
    tion, West African Yellow Fever
    Commission
Yellow fever vaccine, 4, 43, 127-129
Yellow fever virus, 4, 44-45, 50-52, 97,
    111, 127, 129

"Yellow Jack," 8
Young, William A., 52, 112

Zaria, Nigeria, 71